TRUTH
MEDICINE

TRUTH MEDICINE

HEALING AND LIVING AUTHENTICALLY

THROUGH PSYCHEDELIC

PSYCHOTHERAPY

MICHAEL RYOSHIN SAPIRO, PsyD

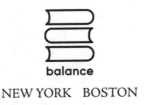

NEW YORK BOSTON

The information contained in this book is intended for use as general information only. It does not constitute medical or legal advice. The reader should consult a health or medical provider in all matters relating to their health. Parts of this book describe activities that could violate federal, state, or local laws and nothing in this book is intended to recommend any action that would cause anyone to do so. The author and publisher specifically disclaim all responsibility for any injury, loss, risk (personal or otherwise), legal consequence or incidental or consequential damage allegedly arising from any contents of this book.

Copyright © 2025 by Michael Ryoshin Sapiro

Cover design by Jaya Nicely
Cover copyright © 2025 by Hachette Book Group, Inc.

Hachette Book Group supports the right to free expression and the value of copyright. The purpose of copyright is to encourage writers and artists to produce the creative works that enrich our culture.

The scanning, uploading, and distribution of this book without permission is a theft of the author's intellectual property. If you would like permission to use material from the book (other than for review purposes), please contact Permissions@hbgusa.com. Thank you for your support of the author's rights.

Balance
Hachette Book Group
1290 Avenue of the Americas
New York, NY 10104
GCP-Balance.com
@GCPBalance

First Edition: June 2025

Balance is an imprint of Grand Central Publishing. The Balance name and logo are registered trademarks of Hachette Book Group, Inc.

The publisher is not responsible for websites (or their content) that are not owned by the publisher.

The Hachette Speakers Bureau provides a wide range of authors for speaking events. To find out more, go to hachettespeakersbureau.com or email HachetteSpeakers@hbgusa.com.

Balance books may be purchased in bulk for business, educational, or promotional use. For information, please contact your local bookseller or email the Hachette Book Group Special Markets Department at Special.Markets@hbgusa.com.

Print book interior design by Bart Dawson.

Library of Congress Cataloging-in-Publication Data has been applied for.

ISBNs: 978-0-306-83639-8 (hardcover) 978-0-306-83641-1 (ebook)

Printed in Canada

MRQ

Printing 1, 2025

This book is dedicated to my first responders and combat veterans who have shown me that true courage is what is needed not just on a call or downrange but also in facing themselves back home. I do what I do for you all.

And to the boys in the 3 a.m. Tribe, the Unholy Sangha. Keep healing, mfers.

CONTENTS

Three Simple Truths — ix
A Note on Sources and Language — xi
Acknowledgments — xiii
Foreword — xvii
Introduction to Psychedelic Psychotherapy — xix

PART ONE
THE HEART IS THE HERO

Chapter 1
A New Approach to Mental Health — 3

Chapter 2
Medicine and the Power of Truth — 23

Chapter 3
Patchwork Persona — 51
Lies and the Fatal Misalignment

Chapter 4
The Next You — 70
Authentic and Aligned

PART TWO
THE WOUNDED HEART GOES ON A JOURNEY

Chapter 5
Preparation — 93
Discovering the Heart of the Hurt

Chapter 6
Truth Medicine — 121
It's Go Time!

Chapter 7
When the Journey Gets Tough   136
Navigating Challenging Experiences

Chapter 8
Psyche and Cosmos   162
Everything, Everywhere, All at Once

Chapter 9
Ordinary Mysticism   179
The Power of the Present Moment

PART THREE
THE HEART IS HOME

Chapter 10
Integration   195
The Art of Curating the Good Life

Chapter 11
Embodiment   215
The Art of Authenticity

Questions to Ask a Psychedelic Psychotherapist	233
Resources	235
Notes	237
Index	241

THREE SIMPLE TRUTHS

THESE THREE SIMPLE truths are the way to healing, good mental health, and embodying who you are meant to be. Learning and practicing these truths isn't easy; this book is an offering rooted in these truths, and they are the foundation of psychedelic psychotherapy:

1. Accepting and loving yourself unconditionally ensures that, for the most part, you will naturally take good care of yourself instead of choosing harmful habits and destructive behaviors.
2. A life of authenticity and alignment is possible when you speak and live your truth.
3. The wisdom you need is within you, now. Feel your body and listen to your heart when making decisions and choosing actions. Your body and heart already know what is good for you and what is not. Living embodied is living fully!

Your well-being depends on you. The primary purpose of this book is to inspire you to speak and live your truth and to be authentic, which I believe are the keys to good mental health. Being fully yourself is not only good for you but also good for your family, community, all humanity, and the whole planet. We need you to be fully alive and to be fully yourself. Stop living someone else's ideas of what your life should be. Learn to listen to and follow your own heart's guidance.

Read with this in mind.

And if this book inspires you to consider, and maybe even engage in, psychedelic psychotherapy, then all the better!

For the sake of all beings and the world we live in, may this book wake up what is dormant in you, what has always yearned to be expressed.

A NOTE ON SOURCES AND LANGUAGE

SOURCES

THROUGHOUT THIS BOOK, I share client stories and transcripts of sessions. I have changed names and used some composites to retain privacy. I am grateful to my clients for their trust, courage, and fortitude throughout their healing journeys.

LANGUAGE

In general, there are so many variations, opinions, and perspectives on terms in our field. I am not looking to coin or create new definitions for terms that are just as elusive as the phenomena that arise during a psychedelic session.

I use words like *mind, heart, spirit, soul, sacred, psyche, cosmos, consciousness, cosmic* and *unitive consciousness, God, mystery,* and *universe.* I, like you, really have no concrete idea what any of these terms actually mean! But I do have direct experience of each one, in some expanded or limited capacity, and most likely so do you. For those of us who have done psychedelics or who have a long-term spiritual practice that we are dedicated and committed to, these concepts have personal meaning. For others, these concepts are mysterious, hard to reach, or unbelievable. All these responses are valid. What we know at this point in the research is that people who use psychedelics ultimately form a new or deeper relationship with the world within themselves as well as the greater, expanded world outside what we call "I."

You may not use these terms in your daily life, or you may even be uncomfortable with them. I will do my absolute best in this book to make these concepts practical and understandable so that as you read words like *psyche, soul, heart,* and *cosmos* they make sense in the context of both regular life and psychedelic psychotherapy.

I take full credit for anything that is or remains confusing and for the use of language that might not hit the mark.

Finally, in my work outside of the state of Idaho, I was not using my privilege to practice as a licensed psychologist.

ACKNOWLEDGMENTS

First and foremost, because Jewish mothers do not come in second, I would like to thank my mom for her unwavering support throughout my life. Though at times very difficult, the healing of our relationship and her unconditional love have made living easier for me. Thanks, Mom! You should all try having a Jewish mother once in your life; it's quite a trip. Next comes Dr. Cassandra Vieten, my mentor, co-teacher, and dearest friend. Without her and her guidance I would not have the career I do. From our work at the Institute of Noetic Sciences (IONS), Esalen, and University of California, San Diego (UCSD), and together on numerous projects, I have learned so much about the transformation of consciousness and what it means to live a dedicated life of service to humanity and the planet. Cassi, I am forever indebted to you.

I wish to thank all my spiritual teachers, including Richard Miller, James Baraz, Larry Jissen Christensen, Gyokuko Carlson, Jan Chozen Bays, Ajahn Sanya, and Ajahn Ganchano. And my incredible depth-oriented psychotherapist Dr. John Berandino, who has saved my life on more than one occasion.

Of course, a *big* thanks to two superwomen in the publishing field: my agent, Karen Murgolo, of Aevitas Creative Management; and Renée Sedliar at Grand Central Publishing. This book would not have been possible without the two of you and your creative energy and know-how.

Thanks to Oliver Wood for our friendship and our early-morning discussions on creativity, artistry, spirituality, finding inspiration in the struggle, the muse, and overcoming adversity with the heart's wisdom. Your music saved my life, and now your friendship helps me thrive in it.

A big, deep-felt thanks to my partners in the psychedelic space. First and foremost, to Kyle Buller and Joe Moore of Psychedelics Today and to the rest of the Vital team: Johanna Hilla and David Drapkin. To Dr. Rael Cahn and Dr. Katherine MacLean for their dedication to and authenticity in the integrated fields of Buddhism and psychedelics. And for my longtime friendship with Valerie Beltran of Zendo Project. Much love to my friend and colleague Nykol Baily Rice, owner and operator of Boise Ketamine Clinic, a place where work gets done well. And to Marcella and all the staff at BKC, where your presence and heart make such a difference for the clients. Carly Doucette, RN, psychedelic psych nurse extraordinaire. Thanks to Marisa Radha Weppner, who co-led several years' worth of ketamine group sessions with me. Molly Downey of Etheric Healing for her ethereal energy work during ketamine sessions and groups. I also taught for several years with Angie Leek of Holos Foundation, friend and wise counsel, who does incredible work on integration in the field, as well as Emma Knighton, known for her loving and fierce advocacy of ethics. Big thanks to my coleader Lara Tambacopoulou as she and I continue to collaborate in many incredible places of the world to offer very deep, nourishing, loving, and supportive retreats. Thanks to the veteran community, including Capt. (Dr.) Bob Koffman, US Navy (Ret.); former Marine Dr. Zach Skiles; Dr. James Muir; US Army Green Beret Sgt. Brett LaFortune; Amber and former Navy SEAL Marcus Capone at Veterans Exploring Treatment Solutions (VETS); the Sabot Foundation team; Dr. Martín Polanco at the Mission Within; and former Marine corpsman Mark Nicholas.

Thanks to director Brandon Kapelow for inviting me to be the featured clinician in his powerful documentary, *An Act of Service*,

ACKNOWLEDGMENTS

which is still earning awards. A huge thanks to Captain Rob Christensen of the Boise Fire Department for the invitation some years ago into the special world of First Responders and for starting me off at Station 5. Without your support, Rob, I wouldn't be doing the work I am now with First Responders across disciplines. Going on calls with Station 5 changed the way I operate as a clinician, and it gave me great respect for the incredibly intense and important work that firefighters, police officers, EMS workers, and wild land firefighters do on all our behalf. Everyday. Nonstop.

Many thanks to Lauren Rose Ludkte, who is my exec assistant, project manager, and wise counsel who helped research this book. And to the rest of my team, Janessa White and Josh Walker, for helping me build a platform for these teachings. I could not have such a blessed life without my sister, her husband, and their kiddos, and my family and all my dearest friends. To my amazing ex-wife, E., whose wisdom and groundedness truly supported me in becoming the man I am today. To my dog, Bruce Moses, who is the most cherished friend I have ever had and who taught me unconditional love, unrestrained play, and patience. To my dad and Heather, who taught me the virtue of service and politeness. To Petra, who, with grace, kindness, and love, gave me space to truly be and express myself. For this and more, I'm forever grateful.

And because I wrote this book by hand, much gratitude to the trees that gave of their fibers for this project to come to life.

Thank you to all my clients, patients, and students. I am so much better at my work because you all gave so much of yourselves to your own well-being and taught me so much in the process.

FOREWORD

For over fifty years, I have devoted myself to mainstreaming psychedelic-assisted therapies for public use. Although the pursuit of health and transformation using psychedelics is as old as our primitive ancestors, we are now in a time when we can share these powerful medicines with our most vulnerable populations. In doing so, today's pioneering practitioners will bring these therapies forward into the future. We need thousands of trained therapists and healers who understand the complexities and nuances of using psychedelics in the treatment of a wide variety of disorders. What's more, we need trained therapists to be "ethnographers of the inner human experience," as Dr. Mike Sapiro writes so poignantly in this book. As the field continues to develop, a host of new protocols and programs will integrate psychedelic medicine into therapy. What I appreciate most about Dr. Mike's approach, even more than him sharing his psychotherapeutic process, is his insight into human nature, the mind, and what it takes for us to thrive.

Through compassion and caring about our suffering and ultimate transformation, he brings us to a place within ourselves that is longing to be exposed, healed, and loved. His focus on truth, authenticity, and unconditional love as medicines strikes at the heart of this work to which I, too, have dedicated so many years. In the end, we are all wanting to heal what hurts and to grow through the challenges of being alive toward thriving. What I have found time and time again is that people who engage in psychedelic therapies not only learn to love themselves but also begin to express dormant parts of themselves that they need to live fully. In *Truth Medicine*, Dr. Mike speaks directly to this point and shares how psychedelic-assisted therapy points us toward an authenticity that he suggests is essential for good mental health. In a time of increasing social unrest and political divisiveness, his message is very timely: Psychedelic-assisted therapy not only heals us personally but also lends itself toward increasing belonging and inclusiveness in our communities.

Although we still have a great deal of work to do to bring these therapies into the mainstream, I am glad to be working alongside clinicians and healers like Mike who dedicate their lives to the well-being of us all. We must respect psychedelic medicines and their accompanying therapies and take them seriously, because the health of our future may well depend on them. And *Truth Medicine* does just that.

—Rick Doblin, PhD, founder and president, Multidisciplinary Association for Psychedelic Studies (MAPS)

INTRODUCTION TO PSYCHEDELIC PSYCHOTHERAPY

ARE YOU LIVING the life you want?

I'd like you to keep this question in mind as you read this book. It's what drives most people who come to see me for psychedelic psychotherapy. Although many of my clients talk about not wanting to feel anxious or depressed, their underlying motivation for engaging in this type of therapy is wanting to feel fully alive, to feel more engaged in their own life, and to be the person their heart knows them to be.

In this book, I write about what I witness during this work of psychedelic psychotherapy (PP) mostly within the practice of ketamine-assisted psychotherapy (KAP), although other medicines will be discussed. I'm an ethnographer of the inner human experience, specifically in regard to nonordinary states of consciousness. I share what I've observed not so that you can duplicate it in psychedelic psychotherapy but rather so that you can learn to pay more attention to your own inner world as a way of awakening what is true within you.

If you are a therapist, know that I'm not advocating for you to adopt my method but for you to take on the role of observer as well as healer during this work. This book is about how people make difficult changes within their own psyche and identify the original sources of their pain and limiting, harmful beliefs, thoughts, and habits of mind in the service of healing and growth.

This is not a sexy book. I do not exclaim the virtues of the psychedelic experience as all pretty lights, fanciful geometric shapes, elves in the machinery, and blissed-out experiences of the universe (but all those things may happen). This is a book about healing ourselves at the deepest level of our core wounds and about becoming the most authentic version of ourselves through that healing process. This book is about the power of discovering, speaking, and living our truths. This process has a cost: The work is hard, grueling even, at times. But it is also beautiful and full of splendor, awe, and, ultimately, love. In the end, an individual might even discover they love who they are—and what a relief and joy that is. Like any arduous journey into the depths of a wild forest, there are mysteries and miracles, meetings with allies and adversaries, lanterns to guide us, and dense fog that obscures the path and causes us to lose our way; fear and courage arise simultaneously. All in the service of healing and growth.

During sessions, I do play in the realm of the cosmos and help people mine their psyche for their own benefit. That said, I want to be clear that I am not a shaman. I do not believe people can become shamans in certificate programs or by going to multiple retreats and then deciding they can do this work. To be a shaman means to be initiated over many years into a healing and spiritual tradition that is steeped in a particular culture in a particular place, in relationship to the land and its plants and animals. Each healing tradition has a cosmology and makes very particular meaning of events, visions, symbols, and signs in order to heal people of disease and to clarify dreams, to name just a few purposes of shamanism.

I am, instead, a clinical psychologist by trade who uses particular medicines paired with Buddhist psychological practices to enhance my work and my clients' healing experiences while engaged in psychedelic psychotherapy.

As a psychedelic psychotherapist, I help people skillfully navigate altered states of consciousness, or nonordinary states of consciousness, for the sake of their healing and personal awakening, which I believe lend themselves to our collective transformation. The medicine unlocks aspects of deeper reality, and my job is to use that sacred material to help clients heal themselves and ultimately to grow. *This is real-time transformation.* Clients slow down and become the neutral, loving observer to all the arisings of their mind and personality. They do this in session by learning how to ride the waves of their emotions and swim in the muck of their mind without being pulled into it. They learn to remain steady in their discomfort and strong when they are challenged. And they do this with the power of their mind and heart and by focusing their loving awareness on themselves and their experience during sessions.

Clients find these keys and clues in their inner journey and put them to immediate use the moment they need them during a session, thus creating new responses to old habits or patterns of thought. This is the power of psychedelic psychotherapy: real-time growth, real-time healing.

With characters like Timothy Leary, Ram Dass, and Ken Kesey involved, psychedelics became the stuff of legend and lore for modern Westerners. Only in the last few years have psychedelics and psychedelic-assisted therapies been accepted as evidenced-based treatments for a variety of mental health concerns. They are gaining the support of Congress, veterans, and first responders nationwide; the *New York Times* is reporting on them;[1] they are trending as a subject on podcasts and in Netflix series; and Michael Pollan has written a best-selling book about them. Hundreds of scientific studies highlight the biological pathways that induce neuroplasticity, or the brain's ability to adapt and change through growth and reorganization, with psychedelic use. Multiple national organizations sponsor psychedelic retreats for combat veterans and first responders to help them heal post-traumatic stress disorder (PTSD), depression, and substance abuse disorders. Directors of recognized integrative medicine clinics are referring their patients with untreatable diseases to psychedelic-assisted therapists who specialize in end-of-life care using psychedelics.

Because of this global shift, it becomes increasingly important for people with mental health concerns such as PTSD, chronic trauma, depression, anxiety, substance use issues, spiritual and existential crises, and feelings of isolation and the therapists who treat them to better understand and be prepared for the innovative use of psychedelic psychotherapy.

How does psychedelic therapy benefit the individual, communities, and specialized groups like first responders and combat veterans? And what actually occurs in a session, in group settings, and on retreats that makes this therapy so revolutionary? Is this treatment right for everyone? If not, why not and who would be excluded? *Truth Medicine* explores these topics from a heart-centered, integrative approach. Psychedelic psychotherapy addresses healing and transformation on a variety of levels, including the physiological, psychological, social, and spiritual. This book includes advice and case studies that are inspiring, engaging, and raw. My hope is that it will leave you feeling uplifted and hopeful about your own healing and transformation as well as the healing of your community.

The core message is that *truth heals wounds and leads to transformation* and that psychedelic therapy is the most powerful and accelerated intervention we have to date to help clients find their truth. Discovering, exposing, speaking, and ultimately living one's truth is the missing component in traditional psychotherapy. The ego and its defenses are often so strong that people continue to protect, project, and even perpetuate the lies they have been told about themselves. Many of our initial core wounds and traumas create beliefs about ourselves, others, and the world that become programmed into our personality as fixed and seemingly permanent beliefs. Even though these negative self-beliefs do not serve us, and usually cause us great harm, we continue to reinforce these detrimental limiting beliefs, which creates fatal misalignments in our lives. These misalignments ultimately are the cause of our depression, anxiety, and existential dread, and they underlie many of the chronic mental and physical health disorders so many of us suffer from.

Traditional psychotherapy is a work-around of this fatal misalignment. It teaches us coping skills and strategies to beat depression and anxiety or to overcome trauma. Rarely does it directly address the harmful lies told to us about ourselves or the deeper truths hidden in our protected and guarded heart. In psychedelic therapy, the medicine acts as a truth serum, freeing us to see and speak clearly about the conditions and programming that have created this fatal misalignment. And it allows us to do so in a very short time. It also shows us our attachment to the very programming we have internalized that keeps us in a self-perpetuating prison of our own suffering. Through psychedelic therapy, we can directly identify the harm done during traumas, and that identification process can liberate us.

IDENTIFYING OUR TRUTHS IS LIBERATING

Here are the truths: We have been lied to about ourselves, and these lies create limiting beliefs that are programmed into our personality. We internalize these lies, believing them to be true, which leaves us feeling misaligned in our life because we are not living our truths and being authentically who we are. Internalization of the lies causes depression, anxiety, existential dread, and other serious mental, physical, and spiritual health concerns. The deeper truths about ourselves, our purpose, our gifts, our worth, and our place in the world must be discovered, brought forward, spoken, nurtured, embodied, witnessed, and shared.

Psychedelic therapy has been shown to be a very powerful tool for accelerating this process of healing and growth.[2] This book covers both the power of truth and how psychedelic psychotherapy works.

In Part One, I detail my psychedelic psychotherapy philosophy, framework, and orientation I use with clients with PTSD and trauma, anxiety, depression, agoraphobia, obsessive-compulsive disorder (OCD), difficult personality traits, and other complex mental health conditions. I also show how I work with individuals dying from brain cancer (glioblastomas) and those suffering from chronic pain. In addition, I share my work with former Navy SEALs, other special operations veterans, and first responders, including police officers and firefighters. I structured Part Two of the book to reflect the protocol I use from start to finish so that you have a sense of the flow of engaging in psychedelic psychotherapy, from the prep sessions all the way to the final integration sessions. Part Three steps us back into the world, and I share how the aftereffects of the protocol can guide and truly change your life.

A DEEPER UNDERSTANDING

Because the field of psychedelic therapy is in its infancy, I am compelled to write this book because the few existing books give only a general overview of psychedelic psychotherapy and now there is need for deeper understanding of this innovative therapy. To date, the dominating theory is to allow the medicine and the patient's "inner healing intelligence" to work together for healing. Though I hold some of this to be true, it is my direct experience through hundreds of sessions and years of leading groups and retreats that the important active and direct role of therapists in this practice is not being discussed or taught at the moment. But an important shift in the field has occurred, and there is an increasing need to discuss and teach therapists how to do therapy while clients are in altered states of consciousness and to inform the public what they can realistically expect from good psychedelic psychotherapy. Evidence shows that undergoing therapy during a psychedelic session increases treatment efficacy and helps sustain the changes made. This book identifies why that is the case.

We all need a hand, "a tire swing at the end of our rope," as Mason Jennings sings, when we are most troubled or when we just can't seem to get back up after a fall or traumatic or difficult experience. We need love, nurturance, guidance, support, and encouragement to help us through the challenges of our life. What's most surprising is that we are the ones we've been waiting for. Truly, you have in you a wise, compassionate, courageous, and understanding self who is waiting patiently for the space to rise, to be felt, seen, and heard.

Psychedelic psychotherapy is one of the most direct pathways to (re)discovering and developing this within you. Right now, which part of you is dominant? The inner critic? The punisher? The perfectionist? The contentious comparer? The avoider? The fighter? The victim? The anxious-attacher? Or maybe the courageous one, the part of you that is ready to do anything to advance your own well-being, is here reading these lines?

The PP process is truly about getting to know yourself, to view yourself in the raw, with no moral lens to cloud your perception. During this process, you get to see all the beauty and glory along with the blood and guts that make up this complex human experience. During this process, which includes preparation, therapeutic journeys, and integration, you learn to recognize and transform the lenses of harsh self-judgment and criticism that often make life difficult and joy elusive. Instead, you may find yourself talking kindlier to yourself and adopting a lens that is accepting of and loving toward yourself, even while evaluating mistakes, fallibilities, and personal blemishes, so to speak.

A mindset of radical acceptance and unconditional love is essential for making the changes you are seeking in your life. You're never going to punish yourself into better behavior. I know so many of us think self-punishment is a good motivator for change, but it isn't. Perhaps it works for a while, in the short term, but it always backfires because we end up feeling worse about ourselves and the behavior changes don't last.

As cheesy as it sounds, love is the way.

Taking an unconditionally loving stance toward yourself has several benefits: You learn to fully accept and love all the parts of you that you've denied, forgotten, repressed, lied about, and hidden, which increases a sense of wholeness and authenticity; and you learn how to support and encourage yourself as you make better and healthier life choices.

I love watching clients speak more kindly and offer more grace to themselves as they engage in this process of vulnerability.

I love watching clients tend to and nurture themselves when hard memories surface and during difficult moments that arise in therapy.

These are signs that healing is taking place in the moment, in real time, during psychedelic psychotherapy. Getting to know and fully accept ourselves and unconditionally loving what we see are such powerful medicine for healing—they create an elixir for thriving.

Have you ever reflected on who is in charge of you, your thoughts, choices, behaviors, daily habits, beliefs, hopes, and desires? Does who's in charge change with circumstance or who you are with? Most of us are completely unaware of the parts of our selves that dominate and control us. During a PP session, this becomes much clearer because you become, in essence, the witnessing observer of your own psyche at work. You become aware of how your mind works, which parts are dominant, and which parts are dominated, repressed, hidden, or forgotten. You also get to see clearly how you are staunchly defending the very beliefs and positions you are hoping to change.

Psychedelic psychotherapy allows us to address and heal, in real time, what surfaces in session, something that can take months or even years to access in traditional talk therapy. Because our usual defenses dissolve and our self-awareness grows in PP, the truth can arise freely. You have the opportunity to be real with yourself, and this is where I find most clients make immediate and sustained changes.

REDEFINING MENTAL HEALTH

This book not only is contributing to the huge paradigm shift in the way we engage in therapy and healing but also is calling for a radical shift in the way we define mental health. Currently, we think that *normal* means "without mental health challenges" and that those with mental health disorders are *abnormal* or *disordered*. Bring me a mustard seed from one household on the planet with "normal" human beings! Being human is difficult, and we all need support and guidance for our healing and growth. I want to move us from the limiting medical model of disease to a holistic, integrated model of mental health and wellness.[3] As you read this book on healing and growth, I want you to think about mental health issues in a new way. As a way to move from the disease model to the integrated wellness model, learn to consider the *root causes* of the issues that present as anxiety and depression, with their array of symptoms. Then focus on what you actually want for yourself rather than focusing solely on symptoms and symptom reduction.

I believe mental health challenges such as depression and anxiety arise in the context of trauma, neglect, abuse, perfectionism, or living up to others' unreasonable and unrealistic expectations, just to name a few causes. These issues manifest as symptoms like poor sleep, low self-esteem, restless and rapid thoughts, fear and worry, and poor eating habits. Although many people do come to me at first saying, "I don't want to feel this way," in my work, I rarely focus on symptom reduction. What we end up focusing on in psychedelic psychotherapy is moving the individual from suffering to thriving, from self-hatred or self-loathing to self-love. In psychedelic psychotherapy, we focus on resolving the underlying root causes of mental health challenges and how the client, as an individual, wants to grow and thrive, and then the difficult symptoms are more likely to resolve. Here are some of the deeper issues many of my clients face:

Root Causes of Mental Health Challenges
- Poor self-care: not showing up for themselves and not even making themselves a priority
- Minimizing themselves
- Shame and guilt
- Unprocessed grief
- Unhealed trauma: living in fear and being overly guarded
- Harmful false beliefs and projecting these onto reality
- Defending the very people who have hurt them
- Believing they deserve to be punished
- Believing they don't deserve to be seen or heard
- Hiding their inner light

What Clients Seek in Psychedelic Psychotherapy
- To express and live their most authentic self
- To feel inspired and to create something original
- To trust themselves and know they have their own back
- To know they will make good choices for their own benefit and wellness
- To believe in themselves and their ability to live up to their potential
- To identify their inner gifts and genius and bring those into the world

To be dependable, kind, and supportive spouses, parents, family members, friends
To be stable, grounded, at ease, calm, and at peace
To be skillful and to live with purpose
To deeply connect to themselves, to others, and to the world around them

When we stop defining ourselves by our diagnosis in order to treat psychological, emotional, and spiritual issues, we can begin to consider the whole health of the body, mind, and spirit. (And, yes, there is a place for diagnoses because they can help us identify the presenting concern and give us a clearer sense of direction in treatment. But let's make this a small place in the whole healing process.) We want to define whole health as moving toward what our hearts long for, not away from what we don't want or like.

When I ask clients initially what they most want, they say, "I don't want to feel like this." Then I ask, "What do you want to feel like or experience instead?" Now I put this question to you: What do you want? Be specific—"I don't know, just not this" won't help you find your destination. Spend time on this question right now. Then, as you read the rest of this book and learn about psychedelic psychotherapy and hear stories about healing and growth, please reflect on and consider not what you don't want but what you long for.

INTO THE MYSTIC

We cannot have a conversation about psychedelics without talking about the feelings of belonging they evoke. Although not every experience or session leaves us feeling connected to ourselves or the greater universe, the majority of people wisely using psychedelics and engaging in psychedelic therapy often report an increased sense of interconnectedness and a deeper relationship with and understanding of their own psyche. I lean into this throughout the book because it is a fundamental part of this therapy, one I've seen time and again. As noted earlier, some of this language may seem new or unfamiliar to you, but it expresses much of the true experience of this protocol.

I use the terms *psyche* and *cosmos* throughout this book; they may not be the terms you use—you may say *soul*, *mind*, or *spirit* rather than psyche; you may say *universe* rather than cosmos. No matter what terminology you use, psychedelics easily provide immediate and visceral access to these domains of mind and universe that are often hidden. Because the material of the psyche and the cosmos inevitability arises in session, I want to explore the possibilities of healing and growth that accompany touching these two domains.

Psychedelic psychotherapy is both deep and expansive. We are simultaneously playing in the fields of our psyche and in the larger grandeur of the universe itself. These levels of consciousness expose us directly to our personalities, our core beliefs and wounds, our strengths and hopes, the interdependent nature of reality, and the fabric of the cosmos itself. Here, we discuss the importance of images, symbols, metaphors, signs, visions, and the like that play a role in our healing and transformation.

These materials and mystical experiences are vital to increase our sense of belonging and connection, which directly combats the often detrimental belief so many of us have that we are alone and do not belong. Feeling isolated and believing we don't belong significantly affect our overall well-being and health and are associated with greater morbidity, higher stress responses, chronic diseases and disorders, and poorer mental health outcomes. We desperately need affirmation and confirmation that we are a part of the whole, are wanted and needed, are seen and included, and belong. This is interdependence: We all matter; everything matters. When these experiences arise in session, we want to be aware of and bring direct attention to them. Exploring the psyche and cosmos connects us to the whole human experience over history and to the natural world in which we all live. So, *what is the psyche?*

In Greek, *psyche* means "soul"; the living essence of a human; the seat of feelings, thoughts, affections, aversions, and desires; the breath that gives life; that which is not dissolved by death; the totality of what makes up the human mind. The psyche has no bottom and no top. In it, our darkest and most vulnerable secrets exist alongside our gifts, passions, and genius.

> *Psychedelics:* A substance that makes the mind and soul visible.
> *Psychology:* The science or study of the human mind, consciousness, and behavior.

For me, the psyche is the integrated living essence of who we are—our dreams, visions, intuitions, wisdom, shadows, archetypes, parts, thoughts, beliefs, feelings, joys, sorrows, wounds, and conscience. The psyche is influenced by our experiences, upbringing, history, ancestry, and cultural conditioning and training, and it informs how we respond to our life in real time. Chapters 9 and 10 explore the concepts of psyche, cosmos, and mysticism as they relate to healing and growth.

MEDIA HYPE AND HIGH EXPECTATIONS

I am so grateful for the current attention the media has given to psychedelics and psychedelic therapy. A deep bow also to the Multidisciplinary Association for Psychedelic Studies (MAPS) for putting our work back on the map in the medical and health field and thrusting it into the international spotlight. This book might not have been possible even just a few years ago without the prolific and supportive attention of the media. And even though as of August 2024, the

Food and Drug Administration (FDA) has not approved MDMA (3,4-Methylenedioxymethamphetamine) for therapy, the show still goes on. Research on psychedelic medicines and therapy continues at various universities and in clinics across the country, and the underground continues its work, as it always has.

But with all the press coverage, there are still some unintended consequences that I must address.

The hype is creating high expectations. People who suffer yearn for a remedy, and so many want it now and want it easy, a magic bullet. In my experience as a suffering human, clinical psychologist, and meditation teacher, the *easy way* is temporary and will not hold. For many years, I self-soothed and numbed through drug use, feeling good one minute, then terrible the next, so needed more drugs to feel better the minute after. (Swap in for "drugs" any behavior you might do to escape, avoid, numb, or distract.) To make long-lasting, sustained changes, I had to learn to tolerate and honor difficult emotions, plumb the depths of my psyche, find and heal the wounds, correct my behaviors and thinking, regulate my nervous system, and integrate all of this into my lifestyle. This is the way. So, when the media hypes the healing and expansive potential of psychedelics, people come running only to learn that these medicines and their accompanying therapy come with challenges and difficulties. There is no going around our pain; the medicine and the therapy teach us to be strong, courageous, and self-loving and supportive as we grow through it. And the universe seems to have our backs, too, when we are willing to do the work.

The hype has created two unrealistic expectations that can seriously affect how an individual might engage with psychedelic psychotherapy: one, that psychedelics and psychedelic psychotherapy are the magic bullets we've been waiting for and we don't have to do anything but take them to be healed; and two, that we will have mystical experiences, ego deaths, blissed-out feelings, and be forever changed. It's true, these things can happen, but to expect them is inhibitory and ultimately leads to disappointment, a sense of failure if they don't occur, and potential blaming of and anger at the medicine, therapist, or the field for being misleading.

By far, PP seems to offer the most immediate, profound, and sustained changes, but it is a difficult road. You will face everything and anything your heart, psyche, and the universe want you to see and experience. PP is no easy task and takes incredible courage. The irony is that those of us with "treatment-resistant disorders" are often the bravest ones, ready to uncover and face what is found and felt in the inner, hidden depths. And this courage alone contains the very seeds of healing we are seeking.

Although the media hype is bringing needed attention to a burgeoning field and innovative treatment, we all must be mindful not to be tempted by magic bullets or the easy way out and not to have unrealistic high expectations. What you are seeking is already inside you. It takes work to access the strength, confidence, and love you want and work to integrate what you discover about yourself into your life.

THIS ISN'T FOR EVERYONE

I also wish psychedelics and psychedelic psychotherapy could be the answer for everybody, but that is simply not the case. As with all medicines and medicinal plants, some are healing and others are toxic. Psychedelics are no different; they do not work well with all bodies or minds, meaning not every person should use them. As the Croatian proverb states: All mushrooms are edible, some only once. Historically, people learned through trial by fire or were led through ceremony by healers: *curanderas*, shamans, and medicine people. Now that we are introducing these powerful medicines into the Western medical and healing field, we must be more deliberate, conscious, and mindful about the benefits and risks and understand that PP is not appropriate for everyone. Rigorous research will help us better understand which populations are at risk and which ones benefit the most.

(I am not saying that science alone has the final say or authority, but research gives us a much better understanding of the risks and benefits of this type of treatment, and so we absolutely should look to science to help us develop this type of discernment.)

There are both medical and psychological risks with all medicines, including psychedelics. Later in the book I discuss these risks in more detail, but I want to give some examples here. Because each psychedelic medicine works on different receptors of the brain and within our physiology, it is important to understand the contraindications and risks of each before choosing to use a medicine in therapy. Some medicines (such as ketamine) are hypertensive, meaning they can raise blood pressure, so a thorough medical history must be taken and blood pressure should be monitored to ensure the client is not in danger during the session. In individuals with a history of cardiac issues, MDMA may increase the risk of a cardiovascular incident and may not be appropriate. Acute suicidality, psychosis, or active mania? Persons with these conditions should typically not be paired with psychedelic medicines because the qualities of a fragmented and ungrounded mind can be heightened or made even worse.

All my clients, whether those on retreat, in groups, or who see me individually, are screened for health conditions. In seeking PP, it is essential you are aware of the risks to your physical health and well-being; ensuring your medical and psychological safety is your responsibility as well as that of the clinic or therapist you are working with. As psychedelics and PP enter the mainstream health field, let's be careful, thoughtful, and conscious about who could be harmed by these medicines and this therapy. Do no harm first.

LEGALITY AND THE COST OF OPPRESSION

In a book about psychedelic psychotherapy, we must at least reflect some on the damage that the war on drugs caused for so many people and for the healing field itself. It is undisputable and well documented that the war on drugs was a federal government strategy targeting people of color, and more specifically Black men, who have been jailed and imprisoned for drug possession at a painful and unjust rate compared to their white male counterparts with similar possession charges. This and the horrendous medical abuse of giving psychedelics to Black women in medical experiments without their consent or even knowledge greatly influence the way Black Americans relate to psychedelics and psychedelic therapies. These are just a few terrible examples of how the legal and medical systems have harmed large groups of people and negatively affected the collective pursuit of global thriving and well-being. For so many people of color, it is hard to trust legal and medical systems that have proved so oppressive and harmful. This matters on so many levels, of course, and specifically in regard to psychedelic therapies because those who may benefit greatly from these treatments may be afraid of the consequences of using psychedelics and trusting therapists. I am glad to see that many of the training programs, such as Vital and MAPS, place a heavy emphasis on health equity and issues of diversity and inclusion. We must not bypass this learning, as uncomfortable as it can be. If all people do not have equal access to these innovative treatments, then the treatments themselves become a force of oppression in the world, which is directly in conflict with the messages of interdependence and interconnectedness the medicines teach.

Therapists and leaders in the field of psychedelics must also represent a wider group in the population. Psychedelics and psychedelic therapies are not owned by any one group of people, and thus the way we use them therapeutically needs to be decided cooperatively and collaboratively in ways that promote the most harmony among us all, while honoring the long history of Indigenous and spiritual traditions in which plant medicines and entheogens have been used.[4] Let this field be a beacon of hope for a future of peace.

Concerning the impact that the war on drugs had on psychedelic use, both recreational and therapeutic, and use in research, please refer to Michael Pollan's *How to Change Your Mind*, Dr. Carl Hart's *Drug Use for Grown-Ups*, and Erika Dyck's insightful and prolific body of work on the cultural and medical history of psychedelics. These resources offer context for the serious consequences of drug policies on the field of psychedelic healing, research, and practice.

The stance I take here concerning legality is one of practicality and immediacy. The data is clear. Psychedelics and psychedelic-assisted therapies are beneficial for resolving a wide range of mental health concerns and diagnoses. Anecdotally and in the research, these innovative treatments are saving lives and increasing well-being for a wide range of populations.

Through the dedicated and passionate work of Amber and Marcus Capone, cofounders of Veterans Exploring Treatment Solutions (VETS), who often testify on Capitol Hill, it has become clear that these treatments are saving the lives of thousands of American combat veterans, who themselves are now at the forefront of pushing for the legalization of these treatments for medical purposes in the United States. Please take a moment to learn about former Navy SEAL Marcus Capone's powerful personal story.

Now is the time. Yes, more research is needed to better understand risks and benefits for more populations, and it is also imperative that these medicines become legalized to bring these powerful treatments to the most vulnerable groups who need help right now. After COVID, specifically, we are in a global mental health crisis, and it is clear that psychedelics and PP provide substantial and significant relief of suffering. We need to legalize the use of these medicines and treatments to make them accessible for healing on a global scale.[5]

TRUTH
MEDICINE

PART ONE

THE HEART IS THE HERO

*I told my head
Why you gotta get so grey
And why you always get in the way
Why can't you just let things go*

*I told my heart
Sorry what I put you through
The trouble is me and not you
You are the wisest one I know*

*Held my breath
Hopin' I could stop the time
And all those stories in my mind
Only a fool would believe*

*Told my heart
Thank you for bein' so true
Now I'm putting my trust in you
Remember to remember is the key*

*The heart is humble
Heart is strong
Heart is the hero of every song
Heart is the hero of every song*

—The Wood Brothers, "Heart Is the Hero"

CHAPTER 1

A NEW APPROACH TO MENTAL HEALTH

Is life as hard for you as it is for me? It's hard being human, isn't it?! I was taught that I would finally receive the approval and love I always wanted after I met some expectations that I later learned were unreasonable and unrealistic. I spent most of my life giving more than was healthy, allowing others to violate my boundaries, which I didn't even know I let happen, and working myself to burnout and exhaustion because I thought that was how I had to earn love and demonstrate my worth. My PTSD symptoms used to get so bad at times that I would find myself looking out the window waiting for "them" to show up, although I was never sure who "they" were. Now I know that my grandparents' horrific experiences during the Holocaust were passed down through epigenetic changes and intergenerational transmission of trauma, which programmed my mother and me (and many in my family) to be on guard and hypervigilant as a baseline.

Like many of you reading this, I suffer the slings and arrows of being human, of living in a body that is hyperalert and jumpy, of feeling dread and despair, and of having beliefs that are not my own that steer me toward living a life not in alignment with who I actually am. I have been working for decades on my own healing and growth while serving others assisting in their awakening to their own truths. To help myself thrive, I practice meditation daily, engage in depth therapy, use plant medicine in rituals and ceremonies, and dance and play with my community; I found my life's purpose in serving others. And still, in the many years I have been serving others and healing myself, I have found nothing more powerful than psychedelic psychotherapy (PP) to aid in transformation.

This chapter illuminates some ways psychedelic psychotherapy is vastly different from and much more expansive in its scope than other mental health therapies. Even the gold standard therapies do not address all the domains I cover in this book based on my therapeutic model. The main difference between traditional therapy and PP is that in psychedelic-assisted therapy clients engage in deep therapy while the ego has lost its hold on reality, which allows the heart to speak its truth and the universe to provide its support through images, symbols, signs, and experiences of the cosmos.

As I will discuss throughout the book, I have never seen or experienced any healing modality that covers so many facets of what it means to be human while connecting us back to our own humanity as the process of psychedelic psychotherapy does.

Psychedelic medicine and the accompanying psychotherapy are changing the mental health field. This therapy promotes greater overall well-being by increasing our sense of belonging and connection to ourselves, to others, and to the world around us. We experience firsthand the unconditional love for ourselves we've been waiting for and needing from other people. And we feel more connected to the great mystery of life, from which all things arise and return.

So many of our core wounds and traumas create beliefs about ourselves, others, and the world that become programmed into our personality as fixed and seemingly permanent features. Even though these negative self-beliefs do not serve us, and usually cause us great harm, we continue to reinforce these detrimental limiting beliefs, which creates fatal misalignments in our life. These misalignments ultimately are the cause of depression, anxiety, and existential dread, and they underlie many other chronic mental and physical health disorders. Indeed, these are the issues that my clients are seeking relief from.

The transformations I've witnessed with my clients after PP are truly astounding, far greater than imagined. I want to be clear, though: Psychedelic psychotherapy and the psychedelic medicines themselves are not magic bullets or panaceas to cure all ills. *Unconditional love and speaking and living our truth are the medicine.* However, the therapy and the psychedelic medicines are vital components in this transformational process. This is such an important point that I will repeat the sentiment: Psychedelic medicine and psychedelic-assisted therapy are not the cures for your suffering. Your own determination to heal, the love and trust you build for yourself in the process, the ability to have your own back and speak your truth, and the attitude of not settling for a life that is less than full and well deserved are the real medicine!

Psychedelic medicines work by giving us a felt sense of belonging and interconnectedness with the greater universe and by dissolving the defending ego, which allows us to feel and explore the parts of ourselves that we've hidden away in shame and fear. The accompanying therapy helps us make sense of the experiences and insights gained while we are on the medicine. *Traditional talk therapy cannot and does not offer these direct experiences. Psychedelic psychotherapy provides a powerful way to expose the contents of our protected deeper consciousness, where our wounds lay waiting to be exposed, healed, and nurtured.*

PP works simultaneously on a variety of levels, or domains, as I often refer to them. I discuss them in greater detail later in the book, but the most basic domains that are affected during PP are physiological and neurological, psychological, and spiritual. Most of my clients report psychological and physical changes during PP, and they also speak about deeply spiritual experiences that mirror mystical teachings throughout history. However, it is important to ground these experiences and reported changes in science, as best we can, on the basis of what we currently know through research.

Just as the neuroscience of meditation has provided us with insights into how mindfulness and other meditation practices increase emotional regulation, alleviate stress by decreasing the amygdala's activity, and increase problem-solving and cognitive abilities by providing greater access to the prefrontal cortex, the neuroscience of psychedelic therapy demonstrates the psychedelics produce much greater neural integration and a significant decrease in the activity of the default mode network, a network of brain areas that is typically active during periods of self-directed thought or introspection. This means we have access to and use more parts of our brain, parts that are normally offline or seldom used, which increases our capacity for creativity and imagination by opening novel ways of perceiving, connecting to, and empathizing with others and the world and by quieting routine habits of mind, thus offering new insights into ourselves.

THE NEUROSCIENCE OF PSYCHEDELICS

Ketamine is the main medicine I use in my work, so I am focusing on it for now. Nykol Bailey Rice, a certified registered nurse anesthetist and psychiatric-mental health nurse practitioner, is the director of the Boise Ketamine Clinic, where I practice. She is recognized as a national expert on ketamine treatment for mental health disorders and has facilitated more than ten thousand sessions since opening her clinic. When I asked her to describe how ketamine operates neurologically and physiologically in patients, she offered this explanation:

> Ketamine has a myriad of physiological effects within the body. Ketamine is the only currently legal prescription substance that

is shown to promote neuronal regrowth and repair, increase neuroplasticity, and improve communication within synapses. The downstream effects of ketamine, which are the changes in physiology which occur as a result of ketamine and its metabolites, also play a role in its high rate of efficacy. Ketamine boosts brain-derived neurotrophic factor, BDNF, which is critical to overall brain health, repair, and function. Ketamine balances neurotransmitters, causing transient and temporary changes in various neurotransmitters. "Feel good" neurotransmitters such as serotonin (mild effects), GABA (moderate increase), dopamine (more prominent action) are increased for a short period after exposure to ketamine.

Ketamine is a dissociative anesthetic, which means it creates a sensation of disconnect between brain and body. On an anatomical level, ketamine quiets the default mode network, or DMN, which is like the reality-processing unit for the brain. It also quiets the amygdala, which is responsible for the flight-fight-freeze response commonly seen in trauma or periods of high stress. By quieting these areas of the brain, the subconscious areas of thought, feeling, or emotions can become more prominent and easier to work with, particularly in the context of ketamine-assisted therapy work. This feeling of disconnect creates both simultaneously the ability to not respond in a physical manner (flight-fight-freeze) to difficult topics and an increased ability to get in touch with difficult or repressed aspects of our psyche that may not otherwise have the opportunity to be accessed as easily in a normal state of consciousness. Ketamine works almost as a chemical buffer between a person and their trauma, allowing them to access and work with traumatic or sensitive topics in a way that feels more physically and psychologically safe to them, creating conducive therapy conditions which are entirely unique in this nonordinary state. It is thought that ketamine creates a chemical meditative state within the brain that is similar to the state of those with about ten thousand hours of meditation practice.

In a more general overview, psychedelic neuroscience research gives us insight into three distinct realms:

- Better understanding of the brain in general, from circuitry and blood flow to how various networks interact
- How adding agents such as ketamine, psilocybin, and LSD affects the brain
- How those changes influence the subjective experience of perception, awareness, consciousness, and identity and cognitive functioning

Neuroscientists, in general, are interested in brain mechanisms and are concerned with how introducing a substance changes the brain and its processes (which affects human perception, cognitive functioning, meaning making, memory, speech and language, etc.). Some researchers are less interested in clinical outcomes, and for others, that is their focus.

I would assume that many scientists are guided not just by curiosity and interest in the brain but also by principles of healing that derive from their work. Some studies only look at mechanism, whereas others include self-reporting and subjective phenomenological data, which is most meaningful to the clients themselves. In an interview I conducted with Dr. Robin Carhart-Harris, he talked about the importance of self-reported subjective data being included in the study because, ultimately, what happens in the brain is less important than how someone heals and makes positive changes in their life.

In separate conversations with Dr. Rael Cahn and Dr. Carhart-Harris, two prominent neuroscientists studying psychedelics and the brain, both made it explicit that the *subjective experience* of the person taking psychedelics is the most important data regarding healing.

This is why I always say that although neuroscience is necessary for greater understanding of how these substances affect the brain, what is most important is a client's own felt sense and subjective experience of the medicine. After all, I am most interested in positive and healthy behavioral and perception changes as a means of creating healing and transformation.

Dr. Cahn agrees and said that over many decades of using biological psychiatric interventions (pharmacology, mostly), mental health issues have increased rather than decreased. Although pharmacological interventions can be quite necessary—your author was happily taking antidepressants for a time—the medicines must be accompanied by lifestyle changes and therapy to achieve the greatest benefit. In this way, companies that are creating "psychedelic" medicines that have no psychoactive properties, meaning they don't engender any notable alteration in consciousness, are pushing Big Pharma's agendas: "Take this and you'll feel better." This model is clearly not working. We must stop thinking that the medicine alone is a magic pill; world-class neuroscientists agree with this sentiment.

The changes we want to make in our lives take personal effort as well as concrete shifts in neurological chemistry, circuitry, and processing. Psychedelics affect neurology in a variety of ways (as do all agents, injuries, sensory inputs, and experiences), but it is the subjective experience of the person taking them—the insights gained, the emotional resonance, the mystical experience, and the sense of belonging and connection to the world—that mediates healing.

Dr. Cahn suggests that the changes in brain chemistry and network operation induced by psychedelics produce clinical differences in depression, anxiety, and trauma symptoms; however, true psychological healing takes place when changes in perception increase self-worth and self-acceptance. Psychedelic medicines don't cause such changes in perception but do make them much more possible to happen within us.

PSYCHOLOGICALLY SPEAKING

We need breathing room. We need spacious silence and stillness to hear the truths hidden beneath the disquiet of our anxious, guarded, and wounded egos. Please take note, the ego is not the enemy. We don't want to kill it. We just want it to shut up for a little while! Like, just be quiet already, please! Actually, in the end, we want to befriend and train the ego to work with us, not against our own best interests. Eventually, it can become our ally.

Until that time, it is usually working, scheming, planning, analyzing, and studying everything, all the time, to get what it thinks you want. It's always creating loops, stories, and narratives about people, circumstances, and situations to make itself feel safe. Its nature is to keep us alive, to protect our wounds from being exposed, to prevent us from being too vulnerable. But it fills the room of our minds, every corner. And the quiet heart needs spaciousness and stillness to share its most precious truths.

SPIRITUALLY SPEAKING

Dissolving and displacing the ego is what psychedelic medicines do. They disrupt the default mode network, and they do this rapidly. Under the influence of the medicine, the ego cannot hold on to its self, and in fact we learn that the ego does not even have a solidified self. It's a phantom in the first place. In psychedelic psychotherapy sessions, we learn that what we think of as "I" is a compilation and configuration of programmed conditions, habits, and impersonations. We learn that our true nature is so much greater than what we imagined.

This is the space in which truth has room to rise. Things we've hidden away, ignored, compartmentalized, and banished come into the light of our awareness, where they can be rediscovered, witnessed, and spoken aloud.

This then becomes the basis for creating a new relationship with ourselves. We first bear witness to our own wounding; we recognize the programming; we learn to tend to our pain, to love on ourselves, to listen to our own heart's values and desires; and then we speak and live our truths. This is authenticity. We stop being the great pretenders, living inside our patchwork persona, and start being authentic and transparent about who we are.

Psychedelic psychotherapy is often about facing our fears; what we are hiding from needs to be witnessed, healed, and loved. This deep, scary material often surfaces during sessions, and so it is best to talk about this early in the book. The end of avoidance, reaching the edge of avoidance, is freedom. It's a kind of liberation from the suffering we are often avoiding. It's quite ironic: We avoid facing what will eventually lead us to good health. The only way to get through it is to go in it. I keep thinking about when Luke Skywalker trains with Yoda. Luke must travel through a dark, scary forest, and he asks, "What's in there?" Yoda says, "Only what you bring with you." But Luke faces himself and his fears, and he comes out trained, in a sense. Or at least starting his training. Many of us spend so much time, energy, and effort avoiding the very pain that can liberate us. Our suffering can be the material of our awakening if used right. But, more often than not, we turn our back on what's causing us pain, and then of course it follows us.

During a PP therapeutic session, we not only face the dragons of our youth, failed relationships, and traumas but also build the skills to do this again with more strength and resiliency, making this work easier the more often we practice it. But before we face the dragons, we have to know we're running from them. We spend so much time, energy, and effort running from the dragons because they're scary. There's dread, maybe there's shame. In Buddhism, these are called dharma gates: The things we're hiding from, running from, avoiding are dharma gates to awakening. But turning around and facing what we fear or what is causing us pain, whether it is actual physical pain or emotional, psychological, spiritual, or relational pain, is so difficult. Every time we turn our back because we're afraid or it's too daunting or we're alone and we don't have the right support, we miss the opportunity to see what's through and beyond the dharma gate.

We never quite get to the other edge of the scary forest because we're not willing to go through it. We continue to carry all the pain with us when we turn our back. We're carrying the dragons with us everywhere we go anyway. Stopping and turning to face one, and looking past its gaping jaws, we see the mystery of the universe and our healing. Our dragons are dharma gates that open to something we might never have known existed—our awakening, our inner peace, our inner joy. This is what we are explicitly doing during psychedelic psychotherapy.

Traditional talk therapies, and especially the cognitively focused ones, tend to inadvertently minimize why we suffer and more importantly miss so much of what it means to be fully human. These types of therapies not only miss the mark but just do not work the way we need them to. Psychedelic psychotherapy is a dynamic, collaborative, ever-changing, engaging, expansive, and integrative experience that uncovers what it truly means to be human. Its aim is fourfold:

- Target and heal hidden core wounds that cause chronic psychospiritual pain in the form of depression, anxiety, and trauma responses that make life difficult
- Help us discover, speak, and live our deepest truths, thus aligning us with our heart's values and helping us live authentically
- Teach us to love and accept ourselves unconditionally
- Connect us to the greater universe, increasing our sense of belonging

These four outcomes can significantly decrease symptoms of depression, anxiety, and trauma and increase our sense of well-being in a variety of domains.

During a session of psychedelic psychotherapy, we are shown which domains of our humanness need our attention, tending, compassion, and love. As discussed in Chapter 5, on preparation, we can go into PP sessions with set intentions, but we must be open to whatever arises and presents itself. Most clients come in seeking relief from the symptoms of anxiety, depression, trauma, and addiction, but so much more is revealed during sessions that allows them to heal the deeper issues that *cause* those symptoms and harmful or unhealthy behaviors. And this is exactly why I have dedicated my career to this style of therapy.

Although not an exhaustive list, these are some conditions that may call for therapeutic attention, at any time, during a PP session:

- Conditions of the body
- Repressions in the psyche
- Blockages in the energetic body
- Stuck emotions, including shame, pity, despair, resentment, anger
- Core wounds
- Limiting beliefs
- Traumatic memories and experiences
- Struggles and pains of the inner child
- Ancestral traumas and conditioning (epigenetics)
- Disconnection from spirit and what it means to be human
- Disenchanted imagination
- Dominating personality traits
- Untended grief

Let's look at the domain of ancestors as an example. The dream of all our ancestors is for us to thrive, to use their strengths and gifts to live better lives than theirs, and to heal the lineage of trauma that has passed down the generations. From the science of epigenetics—how our behaviors and environment affect our genes—we know we are our ancestors and, in a very cellular way, see what they saw, feel what they felt. We learned their hard lessons, which arise for us now as triggers, somatic feelings, and intuitive warnings.

Did you know you existed in your grandmother before your mother was born? You were stored in your mother's egg, and she was stored in your grandmother's egg, and so on. Some of us may have physically and emotionally distanced ourselves from our birth families, but there is no escaping their influence, good, bad, and ugly.

Without doing ancestral work, we are often confused by our reactions to situations or experiences that shouldn't necessarily create such dramatic responses in the moment. This is the epigenetic transmission of life passing down through the generations. I think of this as karma, the rippling effects of our ancestors' experiences disturbing our own waters.

Some of what we face in psychedelic psychotherapy is not our own but is played out in our life and on the fields of our psyche. We may face generations of lived experiences, turmoil, traumas, oppression, famine, and other hardships that sealed themselves inside genetic coding only to be brought out in the most inopportune moments of our life. We need to be aware that these experiences may arise in our sessions, and we should be ready to do the therapeutic work that is necessary to heal what has been passed down. We must do what our ancestors could not.

And strange as it may sound, it is not uncommon to be visited by ancestors who may speak directly to us and give us important messages. Communicating with ancestors is a common daily or ritualized practice in most traditional cultures around the world. For those unversed in this practice of speaking directly to, or being visited by, one's ancestors, this experience can be unsettling at first or even scary. However, as we fall back on the stance of being curious, open, and trusting during this experience in session (as discussed in Chapter 5), we have the opportunity to engage in ancestral healing, which almost always leaves us feeling more connected to our family lineage and ourselves. This may be an important piece that is missing from traditional talk therapies, and doing this ancestral work can have a profound positive impact on future generations (some even claim it can affect those who have already passed on).

Because any of these domains may arise and be present during a therapeutic session, therapists need to have the skills and be versed in each so they can offer useful therapeutic insights and interventions to clients in real time. I often tell my therapist students that they don't have to be masters or experts in each domain, but they should be familiar enough with each to do good work. I encourage them to dive deeper into a domain or two when they feel excited about it or intuitively or intellectually drawn to it. Some students go on to study Somatic Experiencing (SE) to help treat or heal how trauma impacts the body and remains in the body. I direct those who love the idea of integrating parts of the Internal Family Systems Model (IFS). Some students get excited about healing the energy body and go on to study the systems and interventions of biofield sciences and psychoneuroimmunology or even yoga to complement their psychotherapeutic skills.

As a clinical psychologist who works primarily with first responders and special operations and combat veterans, I am trained in a variety of trauma and PTSD interventions (although I do of course work with the general public, as well, with most conditions). I have extensive experience and training in nondual meditation, Buddhist psychology and teachings, noetic sciences, and applied mysticism, all of which I rely on when engaging in psychedelic psychotherapy with my clients.

If you are the client, just roll with whatever experiences arise, be open and honest with the therapist about what is happening inwardly, and afterward reflect on which of these domains presented themselves in session. Take note and start to recognize what is calling out for your attention. This is especially useful during the integration phase of your therapy. Be aware of what is alien and what is familiar to you.

CH-CH-CH-CHANGES

After PP treatment, I most often see changes in clients in the following areas:

- Perspective, outlook, mindset, and thinking styles
- Behaviors and habits
- Personality traits
- Spirituality and how it's applied in daily life

The changes in these domains make a difference in reducing the symptoms of anxiety, depression, trauma, and addiction. These burdensome symptoms really do dampen and make our lives challenging. I do not minimize the negative impact of panic, worry, despair, dread, and fear on our ability to thrive and flourish. But when we heal the underlying causes of these emotional states and make positive changes in our thinking, behaviors, and speech, our reality changes for the better, as does the way we *feel* in our body and life.

Psychedelic psychotherapy has been shown to regulate (suppressing or activating) our nervous system depending on what is needed for balance, expand our relationship with the world by helping us feel more connected and less isolated, and help restore a positive relationship with our body, thus making it easier to make healthier choices for our health and well-being.

Many clients who come to me for healing often complain that their relationships with others are difficult and their communication skills are poor. They tend either to be people pleasers or to have contentious relationships with others, which leaves them feeling resentful and disconnected. The behaviors they notice about themselves in their relationships were generally created in the context of their childhood relationships. In other words, the model for the way we communicate today was built and installed in us when we were very young, and thus, it's baked into our personality. So many of the struggles my clients face in relationships result from the way they express themselves. During psychedelic psychotherapy, clients can clearly see their personality type and these relational behaviors; the patterns and habits of mind and speech that are detrimental in relationships are revealed to them.

Too often, we blame others for the personality-based struggles in our life. Though others do of course contribute to relationship struggles, focusing outside of the self does not facilitate healing and growth. True lasting changes come about only when our attention is directed *within ourselves,* and then we can see our ways of being that negatively affect ourselves.

This is such a vital therapeutic perspective for creating change: We need to experience and observe ourselves while in psychedelic psychotherapy. Our personality and relationship styles, habits, and conditions become so readily observable, it is almost impossible to deny how we create our own reality. This is where I see clients becoming accountable for their actions and the ways of being that affect them negatively. This is also where I see the personality changes so necessary to moving toward a healthy and positive way of being take effect.

When our behaviors, habits of mind, and relationship styles come into clear focus, we can change them ourselves. As we become more grounded in our truth, we feel confident and empowered and see that there is no reason to please or fight with others. It is then that we can choose healthier behaviors, perceptions, thoughts, and communication styles that benefit us and others.

These changes are facilitated by diving into, acknowledging, tending to, and loving the parts of ourselves we most neglect, deny, hate, and repress. In contrast to traditional talk therapy, this all happens while we are under the influence of a medicine and journeying through a psychedelic experience with a skilled guide and therapist by our side.

A NONDUAL HEALING APPROACH

Some years ago, I was sitting in my breakfast nook with my coffee, looking out over my backyard, where the soft pink light of the sun glittered in the tops of the junipers, which were covered in a fine layer of fresh snow. I felt peace and immense joy at the simplicity of it all. Nothing to do, no place to be. And yet, an undercurrent of sadness and grief for the loss of my precious marriage was flowing underneath. With the joy was grief, one emotion swirling into the other seamlessly. *How could this be*, I wondered, *that in one moment of time there exists two seemingly opposite emotions?*

What we long for most—peace, love, ease, joy—can be found in the very moments of our longing and suffering. Although the healing path may be difficult and the daily integration practices hard, the truth is simple: Unconditional love is both the healing salve and our true nature. Discovering, accessing, and applying this love to one's self is the essence of the *nondual* approach of psychedelic psychotherapy. With this approach, we start from this place of innocence, ease, and peace and work our way through the layers of trauma, shame, and untended grief, using love as the healing balm.

Traditional therapies work from the outside in, addressing the various layers that cause us pain and discomfort and moving toward what is good. Nondual psychedelic psychotherapy begins with what is already good and wholesome and then moves with grace, truth, honesty, unconditional love, and acceptance through the layers we are wanting to heal. There is no greater medicine than self-love, so why not spend our time *accessing it first* so we can apply it like a salve on all the untended grief and unhealed wounds that we discover on our PP journey?

Nondual teachings point toward what is naturally whole and unbroken within us. Our awareness of ourselves expands to include all life happening in and around us, including what arises from the depth of our psyche and from the great mystery of the cosmos. This gives us the freedom to disidentify with the suffering of our mind and body as we discover we are so much more. We are, in fact, everything, everywhere, all at once. And in this freedom, we find our essence is pure, innocent, and unconditioned, and always has been. This discovery is healing in itself, and then we work toward its embodiment.

The foundation of my therapeutic framework combines Buddhist psychology and nondual philosophy. This means that I am grounded in and offer therapeutic interventions derived from Buddhist teachings and nondual meditation practices. Buddhist psychology includes concepts and practices such as mindfulness, wisdom, insight, compassion, loving-kindness, forgiveness, equanimity, sympathetic joy, and inner and social ethics. Nondual teachings point toward what is naturally whole and unbroken within us while we expand our awareness of ourselves to include all life happening in and around us. Used together, we can find the freedom to detach from the pains of our ego and mind and body because we find we are so much more.

Traditional treatments and therapies ease discomfort and can reduce symptoms, but they do not ultimately address or target the most significant psychospiritual disconnect that wreaks havoc throughout our lifetime: that of rejecting one's self and denying self-love. Someone who denies themselves self-love ultimately rejects the very benefits of a treatment or medicine because they don't believe they deserve to feel better. This is often subconscious until it's brought to conscious attention.

One of the Vietnam veterans I worked with came as a referral from colleagues at the VA hospital. They told me he wasn't "in compliance and wouldn't adhere to treatment protocols," which is medical speak for "the dude isn't doing what we tell him to do." Of course, he is free to choose what he wants to do with his body and mind, but in this case, it was clear that a psychological obstacle stood in the way, causing him not to engage in his own treatment, so they referred him to me. I spent some time with him and asked probing questions, but he gave only responses that were fairly common among the other Vietnam veterans I worked with: "These doctors don't know shit. . . . They just want to push medications on me. . . . They don't know how to relate and get upset when I swear" and things like this. In general, he might have been right. Trust and rapport are so important, so I spent time just being real with him as we got to know one another.

After a few prep sessions, I asked him directly, "Don't you want to get better?" He paused for a few moments, and then responded, "No, because I am a piece of shit. I don't deserve to live after what I've done." During his combat tour in Vietnam, he witnessed whole villages being wiped out. It was his job after the attacks to make sure all were dead, including women and children. He never forgave himself.

We soon began to address his moral injury. I offered him a nondual meditation intervention for his PTSD that not only helped calm his nervous system but also provided him a window of peaceful rest for brief moments. From this newfound place of ease, he was able to engage with the medicine and talk about his combat missions from a new place of neutral observation that was not marred by self-hatred. Finally, as I hoped, he touched his original essence, which was unstained by the horrors of war.

Nondual psychedelic psychotherapy leads us directly to the source of our innate goodness, which is often denied, forgotten, or buried under layers of shame. It's not easily accessible. But, in a nondual experience, we can simultaneously hold and experience opposite emotions, such as resentment and compassion, sorrow and joy, shame and love, thus freeing ourselves from attaching to one or craving the other. In a nondual psychedelic therapy session, we can experience ourselves as parts and the whole simultaneously, as if we're both the wave and the ocean at the same time. In this way, we do not bind ourselves to any one part of who we think we are but rather expand into our true, unlimited, wholesome nature.

Let's start from the place inside that contains the most important healing medicine and then work through all the layers, bringing unconditional love and truth with us.

A HEALING VOYAGE INWARD

This type of therapy is about taking a fantastical journey into the forgotten and unexplored regions of the soul. Where dreams and reality merge as in a fog-laden forest. Images and scenes appear and disappear from lives lived or lives yet to be lived. We take note of it all. Sometimes during a session, great quiet and space await in which we can explore and reflect. Other times, we are deeply engaged in conversation about what is presenting itself, what it may mean, which emotions are there. Other times still, we may travel back to the trauma and sit in loving, tender awareness of the hurt being done, bringing unconditional love to the parts that suffered the most.

This is a dynamic, ever-changing, ever-evolving and deepening, sometimes frightening and constrictive, action-oriented therapy. We are *doing* healing in the moment it needs to happen, where past and present collide. We are bringing the light of our awareness to the wound and doing something about it, right then, usually by speaking the truth about what presents itself and loving unconditionally. Psychedelic psychotherapy is an astounding therapy that takes place in the realm of the here and now, the only place possible for healing to actually occur.

And if we are the ones to have caused harm or wronged others, we learn to do a type of penance without self-punishment. We offer the same love, compassion, and understanding to the parts of ourselves that can be cruel, unforgiving, resentful, spiteful, violent, and ugly, the parts that act compulsively out of greed, hatred, and ignorance, for these are parts of our humanity too. We love them equally. We grow in our remorse as humility heals us. This, too, happens in psychedelic psychotherapy. And then if we so choose, we can move toward those we have hurt with humility and honesty, and we can put energy and attention into repair and restoration of the harm we've caused. This, too, can happen.

You might be skeptical or doubt that this is possible. You do not have to believe in any of these things as you head into psychedelic psychotherapy. The goal is not for you to become more "spiritualized" or to believe in psychic phenomena and spirits visiting you. Whether you believe these things or not, they do tend to happen in some form or another during psychedelic sessions, so it's best to at least be prepared. Even if all these events arise as interactions between the medicine and your brain, they will seem real enough and you can then use the material to heal and grow. And isn't that all that matters in the end?

CHAPTER 2

MEDICINE AND THE POWER OF TRUTH

Before we dive into the specific substances I and others work with in the field, I again want to make very clear that I believe unconditional love and truth are the actual remedies for our suffering and the foundation of our thriving. For me, psychedelics are substances that have a wide and diverse effect on the brain, perception, cognition, and personal identity. And though I hold these substances to be precious and sacred, I believe the human heart ultimately has what we need to heal and transform.

If we get too hyped up about a particular substance being *the* medicine, a cure-all, we run the risk of becoming attached to and psychologically dependent on that substance to feel better. This happens all the time with nicotine, caffeine, sugar, alcohol, and other addictive substances. There are, of course, times when we need a specific drug for our bodies to function or to help alleviate mental health symptoms that lead to dysfunction. But this is not the relationship we want with psychedelics. What they give is an *experience* that we can use to better ourselves and the world around us, to enhance our lives. They are the raft we use to cross the river; then we lay it aside and continue the journey.

As mentioned earlier, there is just too much hype about psychedelics being the grand cure for everything. This is simply not the case! They are amazing substances that can provoke and provide whole new ways of thinking and seeing while making some beneficial changes in the brain—creating the conditions for us to make the necessary psychological changes we need to live the life we want.

In my work, I make it clear to clients that what we need and what we seek are already within us. These substances make it much easier to recognize the blocks and conditions that make living an authentic life difficult. These substances also help us access the gifts and passions that lie deep within us, waiting to come to life.

That said, I am deeply grateful to these potent psychedelic substances—*medicines*—because they have great potential to help us grow and heal and connect communities across the world by promoting interdependence and a sense of belonging to something greater. So, let's meet these medicines and get a better sense of each one and its uses.

MEET THE MEDICINES

Six medicines are used most often in psychedelic psychotherapy: psilocybin, 5MeO-DMT, ketamine, MDMA, LSD, and ayahuasca. I do the majority of my work with ketamine at a clinic. I also work with psilocybin and 5MeO-DMT with individuals and on retreat in locations outside of the United States where these substances are legal or decriminalized. Unless otherwise specified, the stories I present in this book involve ketamine.

Psilocybin

Psilocybin is a "classic" psychedelic that is naturally occurring and produced by more than two hundred species of fungus. It contains unique psychoactive properties, making it the focus of numerous clinical trials, and is a therapeutic tool of great interest in scientific and medical communities. Research trials show promising results for psilocybin in the treatment of PTSD, addiction, depression, smoking cessation, and end-of-life care. Many traditional treatments for these conditions are ineffective, and psilocybin-assisted therapy (P-AT) might provide a new treatment option for the multitude of individuals who do not benefit from traditional therapies.[1]

Effects

Individuals who take psilocybin report a wide range of experiences over four to eight hours, depending on the dose. These experiences can include visual imagery of multicolored geometric shapes, vivid imaginative sequences, synesthesia (when one sense is experienced as a different sense, as when someone "hears" colors or "sees" sounds), feelings of bliss and connectedness, dissolution of the self and ego, and mystical-type experiences. These experiences are often of great personal significance.

Psilocybin affects neural networks and creates positive changes in personality, increases feelings of connectedness, increases openness, improves perspective-taking ability, improves psychological flexibility, and induces a sense of well-being. Use of this medicine can induce emotional-breakthrough experiences, which are key factors in long-term psychological change.

Administration

The effects of psilocybin are generally felt about twenty to thirty minutes after administration, peak at about one and a half to two hours after ingestion, and then gradually subside in experiences that typically last a total of five or six hours. Dosing depends on body weight, with approximately 20–30 milligrams administered per 70 kilograms of weight.

Risks and Side Effects

Psilocybin has been shown to have low physiological toxicity and low abuse potential when orally ingested. However, as with all medicines, there are some potential risks and side effects.

Many people fear working with psychedelics and potentially experiencing what is commonly referred to as a "bad trip." This kind of psychologically challenging experience does sometimes occur with psilocybin. These experiences can be characterized by feelings of delirium, depersonalization, extreme distress, panic, and symptoms similar to those of schizophrenia. Although these bad-trip experiences are relatively common, evidence shows that the symptoms experienced while under the influence of psilocybin do not persist long term. In the rare cases where psychotic illness does occur, it is generally correlated with a psychological predisposition and not a result of taking the medicine. These findings bolster the importance of administering psychiatric screenings for patients who pursue psychedelic-assisted therapy.[2]

The primary physical concerns associated with psilocybin use are increases in heart rate and blood pressure and gastrointestinal distress following ingestion. None of these physiological effects are long-lasting.

History

Psilocybin-containing mushrooms have been recognized for their medicinal value for centuries. Indigenous cultures of Mesoamerica and various cultures around the world hold these mushrooms in deep reverence. In the 1960s and 1970s, the popularity of psilocybin as a psychedelic staple spread to the mainstream and positioned this substance as one of the leading medicines of interest in the psychedelic-assisted therapy landscape. In the mid-twentieth century, psilocybin was classified as a Schedule I substance, which significantly deterred research on its medicinal utility.

Since then, there have been some significant breakthroughs in the path toward accessibility for this medicine: The US Food and Drug Administration granted breakthrough therapy status to psilocybin in 2018 for treatment-resistant depression, and in 2019 for major depressive disorder. In response, states such as Oregon and Colorado have passed measures allowing for the manufacture, delivery, and administration of psilocybin.[3]

5-MeO-DMT

5-MeO-DMT (also known as Bufo, 5, Toad) is short for 5-methoxy-N,N-dimethyltryptamine. It is a naturally occurring psychedelic tryptamine that is produced by a variety of plant and animal species, most notably in the secretions of *Bufo alvarius*, also known as the Colorado River toad or Sonoran Desert toad. This short-acting medicine has been used throughout history for ritual and spiritual purposes and continues to be of great interest as a tool for psychedelic-assisted therapy.

Effects

Taking 5-MeO-DMT is a huge undertaking. It should be ingested with respect and preparation! It induces a feeling of awe, visual and auditory hallucinations, and sensations similar to those caused by other classic psychedelics. For many who engage with 5-MeO-DMT in a therapeutic setting, it can be a massive catalyst for psychospiritual change. A notable feature of 5-MeO-DMT is the reportedly high rates of ego dissolution and mystical experiences.

Administration

This medicine is usually inhaled through vaporizing or by snorting. The experience is quick, starting just a few seconds after ingestion and lasting about five to thirty minutes, depending on dose. (Snorted material comes on a bit slower and the experience can last a bit longer.) A single dose can have positive effects that last for months.

Risks and Side Effects

Some users have reported an empty or void experience similar to that of sensory deprivation. Users also report feeling fear, shaking, and profound terror. The available data for this medicine indicates the risk profile of 5-MeO-DMT is similar to that of other classic psychedelics, such as psilocybin. There is risk of serotonin syndrome for those also taking antidepressants; certain medical conditions such as fatty liver disease are contraindicated. As with all substances, I always encourage people to undergo a medical screening before deciding which medicine to use.

History

There is evidence that Indigenous people have used 5-MeO-DMT for thousands of years, ingesting it through snuffs. The compound was first synthesized in 1936 by Japanese chemists Toshio Hoshino and Kenya Shimodaira. It wasn't until the mid-1980s that toad secretions became a popular source of this psychedelic compound.

Recently, scholars and activists have worried about the ethical and ecological impact of the increasing demand for 5-MeO-DMT. This increased demand has the potential to affect the stability of the Sonoran Desert toad population from which the substance is derived. There is also concern about the cruelty of harvesting 5-MeO-DMT from toads; because the compound is secreted as a defense mechanism only when the amphibians are under duress, it is argued that the collection process is inherently inhumane. Synthetically derived 5-MeO-DMT provides a potentially more sustainable option to the *Bufo*-derived version.[4]

MDMA

MDMA (methylenedioxymethamphetamine) is often included in the list of psychedelic therapy medicines, though it differs from traditional psychedelics in the subjective experience it provides. It is better described as an *empathogen* or *entactogen*, a substance that creates experiences of empathy, sympathy, and emotional communion by acting primarily as a serotonin-releasing agent (followed by the release of norepinephrine and dopamine); serotonin is a neurotransmitter that affects mood, cognition, reward, learning, and memory, and a host of bodily processes. The effects of MDMA somewhat overlap but are substantially distinct from the effects of classic psychedelics.

Effects

Effects of an MDMA experience include increased compassion for self and others, reduced defenses and fear of emotional injury, enhanced relaxation and sensation awareness, reduced anxiety, and euphoria. One quality that makes it effective in therapeutic treatment is that it can make unpleasant memories less disturbing while it enhances communication and an individual's capacity for introspection.

Its capacity for increasing feelings of interpersonal closeness, changing social perceptions, and reducing anxiety make it a leading and widely supported medicine being researched for use in psychedelic-assisted therapy. Currently, it is administered to research participants and patients with chronic psychiatric disorders such as PTSD, social anxiety, and anxiety related to terminal illness.

Administration

MDMA is taken orally and has an onset of action of thirty to forty-five minutes. The peak of the effects is felt about one and a half to two hours after administration, with the total experience lasting from three to six hours.

Risks and Side Effects

As with most medicines, MDMA comes with risks and benefits, including dehydration, hyperthermia, increased wakefulness (potentially insomnia), increased heart rate or blood pressure, and loss of appetite. Generally, effects are transient and recede as the experience ends. Because it is an amphetamine, it can be cardiotoxic.

History

MDMA was first synthesized in 1912, but its psychoactive effects were not noted until the early 1960s, after which time its use became increasingly popular both recreationally and therapeutically because of its profound ability to open the heart and enable feelings of deep connection and unconditional love for self and others.

MDMA was added to the list of Schedule I controlled substances in the United States in 1985, when it was defined as a drug with a high potential for abuse and no accepted medical use. Although this designation brought many research efforts to a halt, progress was made in the early 1990s when the FDA granted approval for collecting data from safety studies, which revealed no unusual risks and indicated that MDMA could be safely administered in a clinical research context. Since then, and after numerous successful studies demonstrating the effectiveness of MDMA treatment, MDMA is more accessible for therapeutic purposes.

LSD

Lysergic acid diethylamide (LSD) is a well-known classic psychedelic substance also known as "acid." LSD has long been recognized for its therapeutic potential: From the 1950s to the 1970s, it was employed to help catalyze shifts in behavior and personality and as a tool to reduce symptoms of anxiety, depression, psychosomatic diseases, and addiction. It has also been observed that, when administered in a therapeutic setting, LSD could reduce pain, anxiety, and depression in patients with advanced and terminal cancer.

Effects

The psychological effects of LSD are often intense and varied. They can include distortion of sense of time and identity, alteration in depth and time perception, visual hallucinations, synesthesia, sense of bliss and euphoria, distorted perception of the size and shape of objects, touch and body image delusions, depersonalization, enhanced emotional empathy, and mystical experiences. The frequent or long-term use of this medicine can lead to tolerance, but after only a single dose, emotional, physical, and mental stability are quickly recovered. LSD has been shown to exhibit very low physiological toxicity, even at very high doses, and there is little evidence of organic damage or neuropsychological deficits associated with its use.

Administration

LSD is one of the most potent classic hallucinogens available, with active doses between 0.5 and 2 micrograms per kilogram of body weight (100–150 mcg per dose). Its half-life is approximately three hours, but varies between two and five hours, and its psychoactive effects are prolonged over time (up to twelve hours depending on the dose, tolerance, weight, and age of the subject). Recently, LSD has been used in microdoses as low as 10 micrograms to enhance performance of athletes, CEOs, artists, and musicians.

Risks and Side Effects

LSD is a potent medicine and, depending on how much a person takes or how their brain responds, the effects have the potential to create both psychological harm and personal insight. A negative experience while under the influence of LSD can include high anxiety, intense fear, or the sensation of being out of control. Another reported side effect of this medicine happens after the initial effects have worn off: Some individuals experience "flashbacks" wherein they notice their senses altered in a similar way as when they were directly under the influence.

In most clinical trials of LSD, negative effects such as anxiety, headache, and nausea are relatively mild and short-lived. More serious adverse effects, including panic attacks, thoughts of suicide, and psychosis, have been reported in a small percentage of participants.

Patient selection criteria, optimal dosing strategy, and appropriate clinical follow-up guidelines are crucial and remain to be formally established.

History

LSD was first discovered in 1938 by Swiss chemist Albert Hofmann. Some years after his initial synthesis, he accidentally came into contact with a small dose of the chemical and became the first subject in history to experience its effects.

At the end of the 1940s, psychiatrists were greatly interested in the potential use of LSD as a therapeutic agent. It was used in several psychiatric departments in Europe and the United States. The US Army and CIA experimented with this substance as a truth serum and a potential incapacitating agent; however, these experiments bore no fruit because the effects of the medicine tend to make individuals more self-aware and less docile. As a result of its mainstream popularity and association with the counterculture, LSD was prohibited in the United States in 1967. Following this, funding for scientific research of this medicine greatly declined while recreational use and popularity remained high.[5]

Ketamine

Ketamine is notable in that it is currently approved by the FDA: It is commonly used as a general anesthetic in procedures where full skeletal muscle relaxation is not required, as a preanesthetic, and as an agent for enhancing the effects of low-potency substances such as nitrous oxide. Ketamine has also proved to be a highly effective medicine for addressing pain management, treatment-resistant depression, and suicidal ideation, although it is not FDA approved for those uses. The list of therapeutic benefits does not end here.

In recent years, ketamine-assisted psychotherapy (KAP) has emerged as a promising treatment for various mental health conditions, offering an exciting new pathway and renewed hope for individuals who have not found relief through more conventional therapies. KAP combines the therapeutic effects of the medicine with psychotherapy to address a range of psychiatric disorders, including depression, anxiety, PTSD, OCD, ADHD, bipolar disorder, and addiction.

Effects

The effects of ketamine vary greatly depending on dosage. Some of the more notable effects are its ability to decrease sensitivity to pain and create hypnotic, dreamlike, or even fully dissociative trance states. These altered states can be a powerful tool in helping individuals address painful emotions through increased introspection and self-awareness while they simultaneously break down the barriers of resistance that are often present. When used in a therapeutic setting, ketamine has the ability to boost production of the natural mood boosters serotonin and dopamine and help individuals experience a greater sense of self-acceptance, purpose, and a more positive outlook on life. KAP has also been shown to reduce suicidal ideation, therefore making ketamine a potentially lifesaving intervention for those in crisis.

Administration

In KAP, typical routes of administration for ketamine include sublingual lozenge, nasal spray, intravenous injection, or a series of injections, depending on the patient, the therapist, and the treatment setting.

Ketamine is relatively fast-acting and short-lived. Shortly after administration, patients feel the effects, which typically last for about forty-five minutes to an hour. The experience itself is greatly supported by the presence of a therapist, who helps the individual explore what comes up during the session and after. The work continues in the weeks following administration, and integration is often the critical variable in sustaining long-term therapeutic benefit.

Risks and Side Effects
The most common adverse reactions associated with ketamine are nausea, vomiting, dizziness, diplopia (double vision), drowsiness, dysphoria (general discomfort), and confusion. Numerous other potential side effects are much less common, including respiratory issues, muscle stiffness, and cardiovascular issues. Longer-term risks of ketamine use include ulcerative cystitis, impairments in neurocognitive capacity, deficits in working and episodic memory, and addiction.

Additionally, ketamine is contraindicated in patients with underlying health conditions for which increased blood pressure would pose a risk of complications and in those who have shown prior hypersensitivity, who are pregnant or breastfeeding, or who might have an underlying mental health condition such as schizophrenia.

History
Ketamine was first synthesized in 1962 by Calvin Stevens, a professor of organic chemistry at Wayne State University. In 1970, the FDA approved ketamine as an anesthetic, suitable for diagnostic and surgical procedures in humans. It was novel in its application and unique among anesthetics in that it didn't slow breathing or lower blood pressure, which made it a safer alternative to other agents. These qualities led to ketamine being used as an alternative to opiates in military combat situations.

Ketamine use by the public increased in the 1970s, and it was used both recreationally and in therapeutic settings. Although other psychedelics were banned at that time, ketamine was one of the only agents to remain a legal drug. In the 1990s, it proliferated, becoming popular in the rave drug party scene and in the field of psychiatry, where it was examined for a multitude of uses: as a way to understand schizophrenia, as a way to treat severe chronic pain conditions, and as a way to treat depression.[6]

Ayahuasca

Ayahuasca, "vine of the soul," is a highly hallucinogenic plant-based medicine that is made by combining the broken stems of the ayahuasca vine (*Banisteriopsis caapi*) with leaves of the chacruna shrub (*Psychotria viridis*) and brewing the mix into a concentrated liquid to drink. These plants together create a potent medicine that contains psychoactive chemicals: dimethyltryptamine (DMT) and monoamine oxidase inhibitors (MAOIs). When combined, the MAOIs work by blocking the enzymes that usually break down DMT before it reaches the brain, and the resulting experience is often profound and life-altering for the individual.

Effects

The physical, emotional, and mental effects of ayahuasca vary widely, and individuals' experiences are different depending on their physical disposition, general physical and mental health, number of times they have worked with the medicine, amount ingested, strength of the brew, and environment in which it is ingested.

During an individual's experience with the medicine, there can be significant shifts in perception, beliefs about reality or self, and cognitive and emotional processes. Often, the experience is accompanied by intense psychedelic visions, including beautiful visual scenery, geometric patterns, and the appearance of power animals and spirit guides. The reported psychological benefits of the medicine are many, ranging from increased mindfulness capacity, intellectual and spiritual insights, and increased self-reflection to increased awareness of maladaptive behavioral and emotional patterns. The effects can create significant shifts in an individual's outlook and relationship with life.

Research shows that ayahuasca may have anxiety-reducing effects. Other studies have demonstrated that patients with treatment-resistant major depressive disorder (MDD) often benefit significantly from working with this medicine, even just a single dose. Studies also show that ayahuasca can be effective in the treatment of substance dependence.

Administration

Ayahuasca is taken orally and onset of action is within thirty to sixty minutes of ingestion. The peak of the effects is generally felt one to two hours after administration, with the total experience lasting from four to six hours. It may cause strong psychedelic reactions that last four to six hours.

It is critical that this medicine be administered in a proper ritual setting so that users can enjoy the full benefits to be gained. Adequate preparation and a well-oriented mindset are crucial, as is following the experience with intentional integration.

Risks and Side Effects

Many of the problems reported by individuals who engage with ayahuasca stem from a lack of preparation, issues with the set and setting, and lack of integration following the ceremony.

Adverse physical effects include increased blood pressure and pulse rate, nausea, vomiting, and pupil dilation. A tendency toward psychosis or a family history of mental illness increases the risk of triggering a psychotic episode or long-term depersonalization syndrome.

History

Ayahuasca has been used as a traditional medicine and a form of cultural psychiatry in the Amazon basin for thousands of years. It has been a central element in the tribal rituals of Indigenous groups and the mestizo populations of Peru, Brazil, Ecuador, and Colombia. More recently, its use has spread throughout the world, first to urban areas of Brazil, where it was used in various syncretic churches, and then to other Western countries, where it is gaining in popularity for research and in retreat centers.[7]

USES OF PSYCHEDELICS

We use psychedelics in a wide variety of ways, and to some extent significant or valuable healing and growth can occur with each of these methods. Although this book is specifically about psychedelic psychotherapy, it is not an attempt to persuade you that one use is better than another. The four uses commonly discussed in the field are recreational, ceremonial, therapeutic (inner-directed), and psychotherapeutic.

Recreational

For fun! To recreate in the fields of one's own imagination and psyche and in the cosmos. To get high and listen to music, to dance, to make cosmic love, to communicate with trees and rivers, to laugh until it hurts, to bond with friends . . .

In my opinion, adults should be free to mindfully and consciously alter or expand our consciousness as we see fit, whether through meditation, prayer, dancing, drumming, exercise, or psychedelics. After all, that is what we are choosing to do intentionally with coffee, alcohol, and nicotine. To be clear, everything we ingest and consume affects and influences the quality of our consciousness. Some foods leave us sluggish and foggy, whereas others give us mental clarity and energy. Do you consume energy drinks for that "boost"? That's you intentionally changing the quality of your consciousness. (By the way, if there are zero calories in a drink, there is zero energy. Those drinks stimulate, not energize.)

I am aware that anything can be used to excess and become poisonous or toxic to the body, mind, and soul. Recreational use of ketamine can turn into abuse, causing addiction and a variety of mental health and medical issues. Although medicines like psilocybin do not cause physiological dependence, any substance can be used to avoid or distract from underlying emotional distress, grief, trauma, and so forth, thus potentially causing psychological dependence and distress.

Ceremonial

Throughout human existence runs a rich history of spiritual ceremony and ritual in which a wide variety of plants, insects, animals, and minerals found in the local environment were used by medicine men and women, folk healers, and shamans. These ceremonies often involved complex rituals of dieting, dancing, singing, medicine taking, prayer, and chanting. Their purposes were also varied: Ceremonies were burial rites or to communicate with ancestors and spirits, to honor one's lineage, to purify, to embark on a vision quest, to experience ecstasis (a state of being outside of oneself), to experience gnosis (knowledge of spiritual truth), and to facilitate the healing of diseases, to name a few.

In the West, when you ask someone what they know of psychedelic ceremonies, many will say something about ayahuasca retreats in Peru or somewhere in South America. And though these South American Indigenous practices have influenced the field of PP today, it is important to acknowledge that all cultures around the world, throughout human history, practiced spiritual ceremonies and rituals that changed individuals' consciousness for transformational purposes.

Before we delve further into traditional practices, let's spend a moment on the concept of *indigeneity*, which in the Western Hemisphere generally refers to the Indigenous peoples of North and South America. *Indigenous* means originating from a place and may refer to people, plants, animals, or minerals. I encourage my clients to reflect on and gain a better understanding of their ancestry, because the myths, fables, medicines, rituals, and ceremonies of their people may be important as they widen their sense of identity and tie it to what is indigenous for them.

The World Health Organization reported that as of 2023 more than 80 percent of the world's population continues to rely on traditional healers for their medical, mental, and spiritual health needs.[8] Though much of folk medicine wisdom has not been validated by the rigorous scientific methods of modern medical research, it *is* what is being relied on. And so, I want to pay homage to those medicine men and women of the world who pass along healing traditions and to the shamans and *curanderos* and *curanderas* who act as mediums between the spirit world and "this" world and who tackle difficult spiritual concerns. Because there is sometimes confusion around the terms *medicine men and women* and *shamans*, here is the basic differentiation: Medicine men and women use folk and traditional medicines to help cure diseases; shamans help people connect to the psyche, the cosmos, and the spirit world for transformational and healing purposes. If a shaman has medical expertise, she or he can act as a medicine person, and vice versa. Regardless, both practice spiritual and religious rituals and rely heavily on locally found indigenous materials for ceremonial and ritualistic purposes, such as animal parts; plant parts like vines, flowers, leaves, roots, and bark; insects; and the stuff of the earth like clay, dirt, and minerals.

Traditional healing and transformational practices are used for individuals and for groups. Group ceremonies were thought to promote the bonding of tribe members, increasing telepathy, empathy, and group cohesion, all of which were especially important for survival of the tribe, for successful hunting expeditions, and before and after tribal warfare. (We now use group ceremony with combat veterans to help them heal from the trauma of warfare.) Group ceremonies could be for mourning or for celebration, and often these looked the same, but the prayers and chants were different. Group trance could occur with or without medicine when dancing and drumming were the techniques used, although group members may have consumed fermented drinks beforehand.

There is no way for me to do justice to the incredible diversity and beauty of the ceremonial traditions that have come before and that influence us today. If you would like to further explore this topic, there are wonderful books written from a variety of perspectives: spiritual and religious, ethnographic, theological and philosophical, historical, ethnobotanical, and more. See the Resources section at the end of this book.

Therapeutic:
Inner-Directive Therapies and Experiences

Inner-directive therapies use psychedelic medicines to address a myriad of mental, spiritual, and physical issues without much or any psychotherapeutic support. These can include peer-to-peer sessions, non-therapeutically guided sessions, medical and mental health research studies, and inner-directive therapeutic sessions like ketamine-assisted therapy (as opposed to ketamine-assisted psychotherapy).

Inner-directive refers to the interaction between the medicine and the client, in sessions with little to no involvement of a therapist, sitter, or guide. When a psychotherapist is involved in an inner-directive session, they generally allow the client to have their psychedelic experience without directing the conversation or leading the client.

Sitters are those who sit next to or in the vicinity of someone taking a psychedelic. They provide moral support, hand-holding, tending, and care; clean up any physical sick; and maintain safety during the experience. A guide provides the same services as a sitter and makes a few suggestions for how the participant can interact with the medicine, often encouraging them to go deeper into the experience. An inner-directive therapist provides the same services as sitter and guide but is trained to deal with any therapeutic issues that arise in a session. They rely on their clinical training to interact within the context of the psychedelic session without influencing the content.

To be clear, I believe in a client's innate healing intelligence, which works on its own with the medicine. A client can experience profound and long-lasting benefits with all these types of therapies. However, I offer ketamine-assisted psychotherapy and actively engage in the process in session because I believe a therapist's skills, insights, ideas, and awareness of the client's strengths and challenges should be used mindfully during therapy. I do leave time for the client to fully immerse in and experience their psychedelic reality, but this is in service to the work we are engaged in together.

As this field evolves, so too will the various inner-directive and directive approaches in psychotherapy. So, what exactly is psychedelic psychotherapy?

Psychotherapeutic:
Psychedelic Psychotherapy

Psychedelic psychotherapy is a new model of therapy where we work with "everything, everywhere, all at once." And when I say *everything*, I mean everything within us, within the universe, and potentially beyond. We see the parts while recognizing the whole of existence because there are no limits on what arises in session and what we can find within ourselves. Psychedelics open us to the mystery and mysticism of the cosmos and the mayhem and magic of the psyche, so psychedelic psychotherapy includes potentially working with all of this in sessions.

As mentioned, some psychedelic therapies are nondirective or inner-directive, allowing the client and the medicine to interact for most of the session; however, I see psychedelic psychotherapy as including the therapist and their style of healing in the context of the session. As a therapist, I am an active, engaged component asking probing questions, challenging beliefs, offering intuitive insights and compassion, pointing out inconsistences, supporting exploration of psychic and psychedelic phenomena, and teaching useful therapeutic skills during the session, all for the sake of my client's healing and growth. The client and I engage together for much of the session, but there is also space and time for the client to be quiet and go inward. However, clients spend most of the session reflecting and exploring the content and felt sense of their experience as it relates to their therapeutic goals.

The client and I cannot predict what will arise in session, and so we hold intentions lightly and adapt and adjust as the session progresses. One firefighter-paramedic thought he was coming to ketamine treatment for help processing a very traumatic pediatric call, but what arose for him was his need to process the difficulties of being a son of an Army general. He had been denying the impact of his upbringing for so long that this took him by surprise. But by the second session, he could share openly how much pressure he felt as a child to live up to his father's expectations and demands as well as the pain of separation he felt when his father was on deployments.

During the third session, he spoke of the shame he carried for not being able to enter the military because of medical issues (which caused him to believe himself weak and broken) and for retiring from the fire department because of PTSD while his friends continued working. He shared more of his surprise that it was not the traumatic emergency calls that were coming up. I explained that his soul was determined that he heal his deepest sources of shame and self-hatred.

During these sessions, we processed his shame and grief as well as his core limiting beliefs that he was never enough and would never be enough. In and out of the psychedelic state, he felt his pain and saw the conditions and programs he lived by that dominated his consciousness and the toxic way he related to himself. He came out of the psychedelic state lighter and more relieved each session, saying he was starting to see himself differently. It was his fourth session when his heart opened to himself. He saw himself without the conditions he placed on himself, and he realized he had to follow his own path to be fulfilled in this life.

In Chapter 6, I detail more of what I actually do and say in session, but in this firefighter-paramedic's case, I was actively involved in showing him how his limiting beliefs about his worth were directly causing his depression. At first he denied the impact of growing up in the large shadow of his father. My job was to call attention to this quickly so we could get to the work of healing the shame, self-hatred, and untended grief. Because time is limited in session, I go straight to the heart of the wound in the preparation session and in the therapy sessions. I follow the client's psyche's lead to what needs healing and we work directly with all the parts and processes that arise in session. Healing can happen right then, in real time. This is why psychedelic psychotherapy can be so effective.

I believe wholeheartedly in the transformational potential of almost all psychedelic experiences as described here: ceremonial, recreational, and nondirective therapies. However, I have found the most direct (rapid?) method of healing happens when a therapist is actively engaged in the therapeutic process with clients. In this model of psychedelic psychotherapy, therapists are active components.

IT'S NOT THE DRUG, IT'S YOU!

Transformation depends on the individual. I do not believe psychedelics or psychedelic psychotherapy are long-term answers to mental health issues or existential distress. This may seem an ironic perspective in a book about psychedelic psychotherapy. Although the medicines and this therapeutic approach are extraordinary for their transformational potential, we, the individuals having the psychedelic experience, ultimately and eventually must rely on our own heart's wisdom and intuition to find what we are seeking within ourselves and in life.

We want to form healthy, long-lasting, loving relationships with ourselves and cultivate the healing and growth we are seeking. When we feel safe within ourselves, we start feeling safe wherever we go.

When we have our own back, we are more resilient, less able to be hurt when others fail us. When we fully accept and no longer reject ourselves, we cannot be abandoned or rejected by others. The medicine does not give this to us but our own hearts do.

When my clients feel deep ease, peace, and love at the end of a session or series of sessions, I often say, "The *high* of the feeling will not last, but the *truth* you are experiencing will." The hope for all of us is that we end up relying on ourselves when we are in need and struggling rather than depending on the medicine.

DOSE-DEPENDENT

One of the main differences between psychedelic psychotherapy and other therapies or ceremonies that use psychedelics is how careful we must be when measuring the dose in psychedelic psychotherapy. Of course, the dose is also important for psychedelic experiences but more so when we are engaging in psychotherapy. The efficacy of this style of therapy rests on the engagement and interaction of client, medicine, and therapist rather than just the client and medicine.

In psychedelic psychotherapy, the dose must allow for deep therapeutic conversation while the client dives to the depths of their psyche and expands into the cosmos. This takes a very particular dose: Too much, and the client can be blasted off into an incoherent or totally absorptive psychedelic experience where talking is difficult or attention on this reality cannot be sustained. If we are using ketamine, too high a dose can leave a client completely dissociated and unable to talk or put them right to sleep. Too low a dose, and the client notices strange somatic sensations but their consciousness is not freed to explore other realms and their ego remains dominant, leaving clients feeling frustrated with the experience. The loss of ego control is essential in a PP session so that subconsciously repressed memories and truths can be uncovered.

At the ketamine clinic, the staff, client, and I work together over three or more sessions to determine the appropriate dosage for each session. The attending nurse discusses the neuromechanics and dissociative effects of the dose compared to previous doses, and as the client's tolerance builds, the nurse often suggests an increase. The client has a say in how deep or expansive they want to go. And I work with the client to determine a good psychotherapeutic dose based on their previous psychedelic experience or how the previous session went.

An important consideration is dosing so that the client can hold a question in mind and remember the topic of conversation. This is especially necessary when the client is dealing with sensitive memories that they chronically repress or unconsciously deny. The client and I agree beforehand that if these important memories surface I have permission to redirect the client from their stream of consciousness to the work.

If the dose is too high and a client cannot hold on to a question or feels like they are on constantly shifting sands in the various realities of mind, I simply adjust to follow the stream of consciousness that is arising. The most important factor in this type of psychotherapy is trusting the client's consciousness or heart to bring forward what is essential for their healing. However, this is not always the case, as in the time I was working with an eighteen-year-old who was processing the trauma of being abused by a trusted teacher. He was an avid video gamer and we would often have to sift through scenes of *Zelda* in a session to get back to the issue he came in for! We laughed a lot, which was great for bonding and bringing levity to an otherwise difficult life circumstance.

With other medicines, such as psilocybin, dosing is just as important. I often give half a full dose in the beginning so the client and I can engage in conversation that dips into other realities but doesn't necessarily stay there. I give a second dose sometime in the session when needed. If a dose is too high, the client loses sense of this reality and struggles to navigate or direct their conscious awareness back to the therapeutic conversation, which is the point in psychedelic psychotherapy. When engaged in ceremonial use or other psychedelic therapies, participants do not need to engage in this type of conversation, so high doses are reasonable and acceptable.

Overall, there is a healthy range of doses that allow the client and therapist to engage in psychotherapy, and sometimes it takes trial and error to find the border between too low and too high. The best dose enables the client to lose ego control (but ego does not dissolve completely) but retain conscious awareness and enter the psychedelic state while still engaging in a therapeutic conversation.

For reference, the field of psychedelic therapy has terms for these two types of experiences: *Psycholytic* means low to medium doses, done frequently over weeks, and the client remains aware of their surroundings and physical experience, easily engages in conversation, and does not necessarily experience "transcendent" states. This is a good dose range for psychotherapy. *Psychedelic* refers to high doses that cause the client's self-awareness and ego to dissolve. Psychedelic doses are not usually appropriate for psychedelic psychotherapy. The dose I prefer for psychotherapy falls between these two extremes because the information from both states is important and can be used to address therapeutic goals while connecting the client to the greater universe.

When we touch the radiantly loving nondual state of the Mystery, we can then infuse our sense of self with that essence, liberating ourselves from the tethers of our traumas and restrictive traits of our personality with love.

THE POWER OF TRUTH

I was with a friend visiting the Museum of Us in San Diego's Balboa Park when we came across *Postsecrets*, an incredible exhibit by Frank Warren. Since 2005, Frank has solicited and collected strangers' secrets on postcards. He would leave blank postcards in libraries or hand them out to strangers, inviting them to anonymously write their most vulnerable and raw secrets on the cards and then mail them to him. The results were astounding, and profound, and Frank continues to collect and display them. (You can learn more on postsecrets.com.)

More than ten thousand postcards were on display. The ones I read were so moving. Some were funny. Some playful. Some deeply sad and full of grief, longing, regret, remorse . . . and others hopeful. What they all had in common was a raw honesty and a longing to be witnessed and seen.

I felt so moved by this experiment in truth telling, knowing it was what I was going for in my work. I had the privilege of conversing with Frank about his work. I asked why he thinks his project was so successful and what it accomplishes. This was his reply:

> The stories help with change, they are cathartic, unburdening, offer relief, exorcise the secrets out of the darkness with a different perspective and bring it into life. It puts you on a journey where you can come to terms with that secret in your life.
>
> Sharing the secret doesn't make it go away but shows us we are not alone. Feelings of isolation of your secret are an illusion. Secrets are dormant and compartmentalized, but this process and through the liminal space they can begin to release their truth, which doesn't have the same imagined cost of bringing it out in the real world.
>
> I gave people a blank postcard and didn't suggest they connect it to their traumas. It's a blank canvas, but they shared their most important parts for their own release and growth. There's a lot of magic and mystery in sharing one's deepest secret.

This is what I am doing and striving for in my work. The truth heals. *Postsecrets*, like psychedelic psychotherapy, is a process of allowing our truths the space to emerge from deep within our psyches for the sake of our healing and growth. Psychedelic psychotherapy offers people the opportunity to safely share their deepest secrets without fear of judgment, rejection, or shame. Clients are safe to reveal what they've kept hidden—things that haunt or shame them have a chance to see the light and be touched with love and care. This is truth medicine: the healing and liberating power of the truth.

WHAT IS TRUTH?

While writing this chapter, I realized with horror that I would eventually have to define *truth* somewhere in the book, both an honor and a terrible onus. Historically, religious wars have been waged over possession of this concept.

In order not to provoke any theological or philosophical wars with you, and to preserve the integrity of its therapeutic power, I will not attempt to define truth in any way other than as is practical for transformation. Truth must be personalized, after all, if it is to help us heal and evolve.

I find there are three types of truths: universal, spiritual, and personal. Universal truths are those that follow the laws of nature and the cosmos. Everything born dies. Life is a process of birth, growth, stabilization, death, and decay. The well-being of one is dependent on the well-being of all, and vice versa, which is known as interdependence. In a very fundamental way, all things in the known universe are made of various elements and are interconnected by the space between molecules. The difference between us and them, you and me, is actually fictional and made into fact, causing disparities and great suffering.

Spiritual truths are deeply personal and dependent on experience. These truths make meaning of our lives; guide our ethics and values; connect us to Earth, plant, animal, spirit, and Source; and help us find our place in the greater universe. Spiritual truths might also include seeing our innocence, pure essence, and true nature.

Personal truths are relevant to our unique and particular life's circumstances. They can include our values, passions, preferences, needs, and our unique genius that often guides us in our behaviors.

These truths drive us to seek care, represent a deep knowing when something is not right. The conscious mind cannot solve its own problems or understand what causes the hurt, so the soul, which owns our truth, sends messages. When a client comes in seeking change, they usually give so many reasons why they haven't already made the changes. Some reasons are valid, but most are based in fear and shame. Deep down, and as the work begins, clients know what is true for themselves. Their personal truths are what they discover, learn to trust, and ultimately choose to follow in their life.

An example of someone finding their personal truth is the case of a forty-two-year-old woman who came for ketamine treatment to "help fix my deep depression." We immediately set out looking for a misalignment in her life. It turned out her depression was directly related to a feeling of being invisible that started when she was a young child. As most people do after the core wound solidifies and creates lifelong patterns, she continued engaging in relationships with avoidant people, in her case, which reinforced the belief that she was not worth people's attention. During her second session of ketamine treatment, she spent time loving on herself as a child, giving herself the nurturing attention she so desperately needed and wanted then. In her third and final session, she passionately said, "I grew up being neglected and then I found a husband who does the same thing. I finally see myself, and I love her. I'm worth being paid attention to, and I want a partner who also sees me."

When we hear truth, it rings like a bell, clearly and cleanly. "Oh, that *is* true" often follows because there is no doubt. Truth is an internal guidance system. It is felt viscerally. It tells us something important just happened and that we should pay attention.

In Japanese, one variation of the kanji for the word *idea* breaks down to "heart" and "sound." The sound of the heart. The soul speaking its truth. How often do we dismiss or deny what we hear inside, deep ideas of what our lives could be? We reject the very wisdom that we are seeking. Our deepest spiritual truths are often the hardest to hear because they reside under layers of conditioning, programming, self-hatred, shame, trauma, and grief, but they are the most beneficial for our transformation.

The more universal truths we experience and are exposed to in psychedelic psychotherapy, the more our understanding of our place in the cosmos expands and influences the way we experience ourselves and live our lives. The more we identify with and live by our personal and spiritual truths, the more confidently and comfortably we feel living in such a large universe. Psychedelic psychotherapy leads us directly to these transformational truths.

CHAPTER 3

PATCHWORK PERSONA
LIES AND THE FATAL MISALIGNMENT

During our first prep session, Denise, a thirty-five-year-old woman who worked as an executive assistant at a law firm, stated she was always anxious and didn't really know who she was. She had been struggling on and off with harmful eating habits since she was in her early teens.

I wondered if all these issues started roughly at the same time, so I asked her when she began to feel uncomfortable in her own skin.

She quickly said, "When I was twelve and I started growing breasts. All my friends noticed and teased me. My mom said I was becoming a beautiful woman and should be proud. Even the teachers made comments, saying how pretty I was. I had an uncle who . . ."

And here she trailed off. I sat quietly with her, feeling a heaviness in my own body. I asked what she was feeling.

"Gross. Heavy and closed off."

I asked what she was thinking.

"I hate my body."

I asked her to sit with the feelings, to hold space for her pain, and to notice what self-hatred really felt like in her body and psyche. I asked what she wanted to do.

"I want to stuff my face and be disgusting so men don't find me attractive. As I got older, I felt obligated to be beautiful. My mom always made comments on my weight or looks. She would point out pimples I missed, to clean them up or boys wouldn't like me. I believed her! So I spent all my free time trying to make myself look beautiful. I'd spread out magazines with pictures. I spent hours at the pharmacy looking at makeup. I started eating worse and worse to lose weight, and then I would stuff myself till I was sick."

I asked who that girl was under all those behaviors, thoughts, and conditions.

"She was a sweet girl, just wanted to be loved."

And here she started crying. When that passed, I asked what she wanted.

"I just want to feel good being me. I want to love who I see in the mirror. I don't want to put on some kind of costume to be loved or liked by others."

And this began our journey together to reclaim her innocence and authenticity.

This chapter details the psychological impact and consequences of living a misaligned life. Many features of our personality were created early on in response to others' beliefs, judgments, and opinions of us. During psychedelic psychotherapy, we often realize that we are living lives programmed and determined by others' beliefs. I call this living as a patchwork persona. Living inside a patchwork persona can be deadly for the human soul. Keep this in mind as you learn more about the benefits of this type of therapy.

From birth, you have been told messages—positive, negative, and neutral—about yourself and your intrinsic value by the culture you live in, your parents, family, friends, teachers, clergy, community members, and the media. You have been unintentionally and sometimes intentionally lied to about who you are or should be and what expectations you must meet to be accepted and loved. And, for the most part, we believe these lies because don't our parents or teachers know what they are talking about?

Really, any opinion, judgment, or belief someone else has about you is really about them, not you. This is very important to understand because we are trained from birth to believe others' opinions of us as truth, and these false beliefs become the bars and bricks of our prison cell. We are under such pressure to live up to others' expectations and ideas of who we are supposed to be. When we believe others' opinions and thoughts about us are true, we deny what is actually true for us. As discussed later, they become the "patches" you wear.

Here are some examples of patches, others' opinions that clients have internalized and been hurt, pressured, and confused by:

> "You're so smart, why are you making so much trouble?"
> "You're going to be so successful."
> "You're so talented, why are you wasting your time reading all the time?"
> "You are worthless, just like your mom."
> "You're so fat, who is going to want to be friends with you?"
> "You are not really good at that, are you?"
> "I wish you weren't born."
> "Did your mom and I ever tell you we actually didn't want children?"
> "Stop crying. Be a man."
> "You were such a surprise when I had you, you saved my life."
> "Your dad left because of you."
> "Proper girls should not concern themselves with things like that."
> "You deserve exactly what happened to you."
> "Have you seen your face? You won't make it in acting."

"You know you're not that attractive, right?"

"You're not good enough to be on the team, so I wouldn't waste your time trying out."

"Don't ever stop being pretty!"

On and on and on. Painful to read, aren't they?

These messages are everywhere, in TV shows and commercials, movies and magazines, history books and lessons. These messages about people's worth are based on status and class, wealth and education, occupation, skin color, gender, sexuality, religion, and body type. These messages make imprints on children, who then waste so much life force and mental energy trying to be, look, seem, and achieve what they are conditioned and convinced to think is best. This process starts early, and the result is that we as a species have become conditioned caricatures of characters created by consensus. We are caught in an untender trap.

This is how patchwork personas are born: in our pursuit of being just like the characters we idolize or wanting to be accepted and loved by the people who take care of us. We ultimately become a caricature of these made-up characters, which creates the misalignments that cause so much depression, anxiety, and existential distress in our lives.

We are all subject to this manipulation of our character, and it is a death sentence to the soul's originality and innate natural beauty. We are all beautiful just as we are. If you don't believe me or see this within yourself, maybe psychedelic psychotherapy is for you. If you feel like you're living someone else's life, then psychedelic psychotherapy might be for you.

Come strip the layers away and take those patches off (that don't actually exist). Witness what is within you, that which has never been tarnished, that which is never inadequate.

The alternative sucks. Living inside a caricature of a character that has nothing to do with you? No thanks.

Psychedelic psychotherapy helps us take a closer look at the characters, avatars, and personas we are playing and the fictions we are acting in. During PP sessions, those personas cannot hold shape or stay dominant. Their patches ultimately dissolve into stardust because they were never real to begin with.

> Please spend a few moments reflecting on any messages you received or that were implied as you grew up. Maybe write them down in your journal, and reflect on how you feel about them and any impact they have had on your life.

Some messages are direct; others are learned by omission. Not being loved unconditionally hurts deeply. Not being seen, heard, validated, supported, or encouraged leaves marks of shame and uncertainty about our worth. These messages also create patches we wear that influence the way we see ourselves and operate in the reality that we in fact are generating.

Not only do we tend to believe these lies, we internalize all these messages about who we are and drive ourselves crazy trying to meet demands and standards that are not our own. Sometimes we sabotage ourselves and keep failing just to prove these messages are true! How crazy is that?! To cause ourselves to fail to prove true a terribly destructive and false truth created by someone else's ignorance? This is the fatal misalignment that causes so much depression, shame, anxiety, resentment, and self-hatred that so many of us struggle with. We are creating and living inside versions of ourselves based on others' expectations, demands, and harmful beliefs. We often find we're living someone else's life in a body that feels unfamiliar and alien to us.

Some messages are placed on you from birth because of the culture you were born into. How many patches are you already wearing from birth just being a woman, gay, a person of color? Imagine how many patches are put onto our bodies during elementary school, throughout adolescence, during our twenties, and so on. We wear so many patches that soon we are covered in them and our personalities change to accommodate them. We develop a patchwork persona, a false personality that we project outward and inwardly think is us. These personas are who relates to others for us, make choices for us in what we do for work, who we choose to be with, how we interact with the external world.

We think, speak, act, and believe what has been demanded of and taught to this patchwork persona. We cannot feel aligned with our own true heart or original personality because we are living our life as someone else because we internalized all the lies and messages told to us about ourselves. Can you see this patchwork persona, like an avatar you live inside, leaving you feeling completely disconnected from who you truly are?

I remember when I discovered and dissolved one of the biggest, most energy-consuming patches I had. A dear friend and I went into the forest around Bend, Oregon, for a sacred brothers' weekend, where we would meditate, journey together, grieve and support one another's losses and struggles, mountain bike, dance, and camp. Neither of us is a regular marijuana smoker, but we do engage in the ceremonial use of this plant when out in the forest together. We set our intentions for the weekend, offered our gratitude for the land we were on, the people who were stewards long before we arrived, and the trees and animals that were peacefully living there.

After some time acclimating to the changes in our consciousness, noting the slowing of time, the movement of ants, the expanded sensory awareness of our environment that included feeling the vibrancy of life around us, and taking a long, silent walk through the silent, still trees, we returned to camp and went inward.

The insights started flooding me. I saw an image of my calendar, which was often full from one end of the week to the other and had been for years. My body tensed and chest tightened with a visceral pressure. This thought arose like a blaring work-shift horn: "What am I doing out here? I should be working." Which part of me said this and where did this intense pressure come from? Not moved by this experience, and staying still, I asked myself, "What do you want for me?" It responded, "To show you're not lazy, that you are working hard." But that was evident, wasn't it? I already knew how hardworking I was. "Who needs to see this?" I asked. "Dad," who was no longer in the picture. I was working myself to burnout to prove myself to someone who wasn't even there. Fuuuuuck that!

And it all became clear instantaneously. All that pushing myself, pursuing achievements, working myself beyond reason (which affected my marriage) just to appease my father and receive his approval. What I wanted most was to be loved unconditionally, but there were conditions; a losing arrangement for both of us.

I speak several languages, have three advanced degrees, served in AmeriCorps and the Peace Corps, am an ordained Zen monk and poet, work with special operations veterans, SWAT team operators, police officers, firefighters, and wildland firefighters, on and on. Did I do all this for him? No, but the incessant drive to be enough and the pressure that fueled some of my life's work did.

I saw a great black hole on my chest.
I saw my father placing it on me as a child.
He said fill this and then I will love you,
So, I kept filling it, but it was bottomless.
I moved to strip it from me and realized,
there was no hole, and there never was.

Our patches are not permanent, and in fact, they don't exist. But even illusions, shadows, and mirages have an impact, like dreams and memories do. Our personality is formed around the messages we receive and then internalize. So much of psychedelic psychotherapy helps us discover and dissolve these conditions, the various patches placed on us that form the personas we wear.

> ### PATCHWORK PERSONA
> ### PERSONAL REFLECTION
>
> I'd like to offer you a chance to reflect on your own patchwork persona.
> - On a whole piece of paper, draw a figure of your body covered in various-sized patches. Leave enough room in the patches so you can scribble some words or phrases.
> - Reflect for a few minutes about the different messages you received about yourself from parents, caregivers, teachers, friends, strangers, clergy, the media, and the culture in which you grew up. Reflect on the messages you have been telling yourself about yourself. These can be positive, negative, neutral, harmful, hurtful, endearing, or encouraging.
> - Add the messages into the patches until most or all are filled.
> - Spend a few moments looking over your image, making sure nothing is missing.
> - Notice any internal responses or reactions, feelings, emotions, sensations, thoughts, or insights.
> - In your journal, please respond to this prompt: How has your life been shaped by these messages? How have you changed yourself to accommodate, prove or disprove, live up to or fail these messages?
> - Imagine most of these are not true. Imagine taking these patches off. What does your heart imagine lies beneath?
> - On another piece of paper, redraw your body, this time without patches, and place one big heart in the middle.

> Add words and phrases about yourself that you know or desire to be true, that speak to your original essence and unconditioned soul. See yourself clearly without judgment or criticism. Notice how you feel and any internal reactions. It's okay if you don't know what to write yet. If that is the case, also notice how you feel and any internal reactions.
>
> May this be the start of a new path of self-discovery and self-love for each of you who complete this assignment.

EXCAVATING

When I begin working with a client, I immediately look for this misalignment or the harmful messaging they've internalized because these are the deepest sources of psychological and emotional pain. In the first preparatory session, I want to excavate what is under the depression, anxiety, trauma, disordered thinking, dysfunctional behaviors, and existential distress. I often find self-hatred, self-loathing, and low self-worth that come from trying to live a life that is defined by the conditions set by others. And these conditions are usually created by others' maladaptive and limiting beliefs, meaning we are trying to live up to the expectations of someone else's shadow. Think about that for a moment.

The way you push yourself so hard to succeed.

The way you punish yourself for failing.

The way you shame yourself for your behaviors.

These are all mirrors of how someone else treated you and taught you to think about yourself, and it's all based on *their* beliefs about themselves! They whipped themselves, then you, and then gave you the whip, which you are now using on yourself willingly! We all do this.

FOLLOWING THE FIRE

He came in tired, really tired, and had a sadness written all over his face. He said he hadn't felt joy in a long time and that most things he used to love just didn't bring him happiness anymore. He loved his life and was grateful for everything in it but just didn't feel good and lacked motivation. As a captain in the fire department and career paramedic, he had seen and done a lot, and I wondered if the calls he went on were finally getting to him. Because many firefighters have a side hustle, a second job or business they run during their four-day break, I asked if he worked a little on the side. He owned and ran a very successful business and had worked an average of eighty to ninety hours a week for over twenty years! Alarm bells rang loudly in my head, and I started following that fire. Of course, we addressed issues of work-related stress and burnout, but what was more important was uncovering the drive he felt that pressured him to work that hard for that long with minimal breaks.

Throughout our prep sessions, we got closer to discovering why he pushed himself to exhaustion and into depression. We found that during his childhood, growing up in a strictly religious household and community constrained his sense of self into a small box in which he lived uncomfortably until he broke away to "do my own thing, by myself."

We found threads of not feeling good enough in his family and religious community, so he excelled in sports to prove himself. Yet, the deepest wounds remained hidden.

It wasn't until our second ketamine session when we discovered the root of his sadness, which caused him to drink, overwork, and stay in a toxic marriage for far too long. His intention for this session had been to forgive himself for staying in the marriage and continuing some other self-punishing behaviors. He also wanted to understand why he drank so much in the past and continued to overwork. Here is an excerpt from this session, with my comments in parentheses:

I thought I've always enjoyed being alone and having peace by myself. This might not be the case. (It may be underneath, but you've always distracted yourself by overworking and drinking, and now you are not, so a lot is rising up in your awareness.)

There's a correlation between this and the alcoholism.

I'm right at the edge of being able to push through.

(Relax, trust yourself, it's in there. Go toward what needs healing, the pain, what you've been avoiding. Using alcohol and overworking are very similar strategies.)

Yes, to numb myself and to avoid dealing with what I don't know, though.

(Go to where the pain is.)

Just felt an immense amount of pain right here [*points to right side of abdomen*] and went into the pain, but now there is nothing there.

(What are you avoiding? What belief do you have that made you want to drink the way you did?)

And numb myself?

(Yeah.)

Inadequacy. Not enough. It doesn't matter what I do or how hard I try, it's never good enough. For whom, though?

(It starts very young and carries forward in all relationships, or most. It's taught and internalized.)

Seventh grade, sitting next to the girl I really like. She's telling me you're nice *but*, you know, you're not attractive.

(Damn!)

You're a nice person, but girls aren't gonna like you.

(How did you feel then?)

Crushed.

(How did this affect your belief system about yourself?)

Subconsciously, I wouldn't put myself out there 'cause I didn't want to get rejected like that again.

(What are you feeling right now?)

I want to let that go.

(What does he need to heal?)

He needs . . . love.

(Give it to him. Go back to that desk, give him what he needs.)

I'm giving him love. Telling him that he's gonna be just fine.

(How is he?)

He seems a little lost.

(Guide him, tell him more about you and your life. Let him know all the adventures that are coming, the wild life you have.)

He just smiled.

It's so crazy how just two sentences can affect someone's life so much for so long, and the other person may or may not even know there's any impact. And that seed is planted, and that's my normal, and now I'm convinced no one is really gonna like me 'cause I'm told that in seventh grade. And my ex-wife finds that programming and latches onto it because that little seed was planted then, and it affects everything else.

"I'm not attractive." "I'm not this." Xyz.

I have to earn it, I can't just be, I have to perform and do all these things, 'cause this little seed planted in seventh grade grows and grows.

Even though I know it's not true and not reality, I can't uproot it and get it out of my brain.

(You can certainly love him and you, and teach yourself differently. This is an internalized lie.)

Yeah, thank you. That's exactly what it is.

And it hurt so much that I didn't feel it hurt.

(Yeah, it was like water to a fish. Say more about not even knowing it hurt.)

She even said, "No one is going to fall in love with you, no one is even going to like you." Fuck. It was almost like a spell, magic. Man, the ripple effect.

(Isn't this amazing, what you've discovered?)

It is. I don't feel bitterness or anger toward her. The power we have with our words. Oh my God.

(Is there any connection between being told these things as a child and your drinking, overworking, and staying in a very harmful marriage?)

Yes, I didn't want to feel that pain. Alcohol and work helped numb that pain instead of me feeling the pain. I want to go there.

(Good, let's.)

Why did I feel I had to numb that pain instead of being able and willing to feel it?

(Great reflection. So many people spend their lives avoiding looking at these things at all cost.)

Pain hurts, but that's all it is. Why haven't I been willing to look at it?

(Yes, it's not just pain, it's a harmful, hurtful message about your core sense of self, and at that age you're so vulnerable to be influenced. It's so hard to look at that. It takes courage.)

Yes, it does, but I'm doing it now.

(And you want to forgive yourself? This is the start of that. Understanding the context, what happened, where the pain came from. This builds compassion and makes it easier to understand yourself and your behaviors.)

This was a very powerful session for him. He was amazed at what he discovered within himself and how he had internalized someone else's opinions of him. He was incredulous that something seemingly so small and insignificant could have such a powerful effect on his psyche for much of his life. Yet, he built a persona around this wound, ended up drinking heavily to numb the pain, and worked himself into exhaustion trying to prove he is worthy—all detrimental to his health and well-being, not to mention such a joy kill! Just recognizing this was liberating and relieving. He could now spend time loving on that part of himself that was so deeply hurt by that girl's comments, which he took to heart and still carried around nearly thirty years later. Then the treatment began to focus directly on him learning to love and offer himself compassion, which is the start of forgiveness and moving on.

Seeing ourselves clearly is such good medicine.

FROM "SERIOUS ED" TO "AUTHENTIC ED"

Another patient, a man in his mid-thirties, came for ketamine treatment to reduce his drinking. During our preparation session, he quickly realized that he was drinking to numb the pain of his rage, hurt, grief, and sadness caused by childhood traumas. One memory stood out in that session: He was being whipped so hard by his father that his body bounced on the bed mattress and then was turned over and struck on the other side only to bounce again. During the retelling of this memory, he experienced many distressing sensations and internal reactions, what could be labeled *trauma responses*. He had not noticed these feelings before, and when I asked what he wanted to do at that moment, he responded with, "Numb them." The connection of his trauma to PTSD symptoms and his drinking became clear.

During his second ketamine session, he finally allowed himself to feel the pain of that boy. Then he saw himself as a teenager who started drinking in response to his father's behaviors. He saw how he formed a persona that was protective, serious, and angry. At fifteen years of age, he rejected his parents' authority and parenting rights and took control of his life. He did not trust others to have his best interest in mind and quickly became overly self-dependent and isolative. He named this persona "Serious Ed."

"It became my default mode of operating. I stopped having fun and saw everything as an obligation and responsibility. I rarely smiled."

Serious Ed filled his consciousness, dominated his personality. I asked what fueled Serious Ed, and he replied, "Self-rejection, the need to prove myself, self-hatred. . . . I will go until I break." Serious Ed saw the world as all work, serious responsibilities, and obligations and saw others as weak and distrustful. There was no time to play, which hurt him the most as a father who was struggling to bond with and relate to his children. During the ketamine sessions, he recognized how dominating Serious Ed was in his personality and began to feel a sense of freedom and peace he had not known before. He had space and some ease just by becoming more aware.

In his final ketamine session, he saw his core self before it was wounded, and it was good and wholesome. He cried when he realized that before his traumas occurred he was innocent and pure. Living a life inside the consciousness of Serious Ed caused him to forget his original essence.

In our integration session, which began after the completion of the psychedelic psychotherapy sessions, I said, "When you realize you are good enough, Serious Ed has no fuel left."

"If that wasn't there," he said, "I wouldn't feel all these constricting emotions and my default would be one of peace and ease."

As we continued to work together in the integration phase, we focused a lot on shifting out of Serious Ed and taking off the patches that covered his good, innocent soul. He asked, "If Serious Ed is not my default anymore, who is?" This is one of my favorite questions! It brings us to the edge of the unknown, where we have space, freedom, and the personal autonomy to be or become who we actually are. This is the moment I wait for in the psychedelic psychotherapeutic process. Who, then, do you want to be?! Who do you want in charge of your consciousness, behaviors, thoughts, actions?

"Do I just create another persona? A better one?" he asked.

"I don't think so," I replied. "What or who in you is original, without conditions?"

"I always saw people living out their passions and never understood why I wasn't." After a pause, he looked at me and said, "Authentic Ed."

"And what drives him?" I asked.

"My soul does, the essence of who God made me."

"Yes, exactly!" I almost shouted. "And what are his qualities?"

"Honor, kindness, honesty, humility, and playfulness."

"Now you get to practice embodying Authentic Ed."

And he has been.

TRUTH IS MEDICINE

Discovering and recognizing truth, speaking it out loud, and learning to live by it is the medicine your heart has been seeking. And psychedelic psychotherapy seems to be the quickest way to learn to speak and live by your truth. Under the medicine's influence, the ego tends to dissolve or come and go, and its defenses are no longer fortified or held. This means that when I ask questions about those misalignments or trauma memories, the client can no longer rely on their ego to defend, to manipulate, or to outright lie to protect themselves from having to say the truth.

This sentiment occurs frequently: "Oh, my [parent/sibling/spouse/friend/colleague] is a good person; they really didn't mean to hurt me." I hear this all the time at the beginning of a session. And sometime in that very session, the client will literally yell, "I hate my [parent/sibling/spouse/friend/colleague]! She was fucking awful to me!" And I say, "Good, tell me more. Keep going. Let it be seen. Let that out. Give yourself permission to speak your truth." And they do.

This is often the part of the session when my client sees the programming and the patches. We then move from their true feelings and thoughts down to what the actual experience was like as a child. One client had named her persona "Bad Rita." This particular client moved from "I am so angry I was treated that way" to "I wasn't seen, it was like I didn't exist at all. Once my dad left, it was all about my mother, and I was left alone. I felt like I didn't matter to her, so I did all these stupid things [promiscuity and drug use] to get her attention. I hated myself for it but couldn't stop."

"What did you learn about yourself during this time?" I asked.

"There was nothing I could do that was enough to get her attention and love," she replied.

"So, what did that leave you believing about yourself?"

"I wasn't enough," she said. This was a huge patch for her that covered most of her heart and influenced her life in so many ways.

This might sound like a routine discovery that can happen in traditional talk therapy, and it can. But this was our first session. She spoke a truth she'd never admitted before, and then we rapidly identified and uncovered a core limiting belief that was deeply woven into a persona she lived within and that disrupted her life. During the second session, we practiced self-compassion and she learned how to love that wounded little girl. She came into our third and final session feeling safe, heard, seen (by herself, most importantly), and from this place of peace she started truly loving herself. She discovered within her that which was already whole and unbroken. In that session, she saw her son, whom she loves passionately, and turned her unconditional love for her son inward. Here is a snippet of a transcript from one ketamine session (my responses are in parentheses):

Oh my son. He's so beautiful. He's so extraordinary. God, that boy is magic. I want him to know.

(Is there any way to see yourself this way?)

I'm beautiful.

(Is there any way you can see yourself through these eyes, the way you see him? You need to see yourself through a mother's unconditional love, the love you always wanted, but never had.)

Yes, please. It always comes back to love. I am love. I am so loved.

(See yourself in all your beauty, strength, foibles, weaknesses, struggles. She's been waiting for you.)

She's beautiful and extraordinary.

Her Bad Rita persona, covered in "I'm not good enough," "slut," and "no-good burnout" patches, caused her to sabotage many relationships throughout her life because she did not feel worthy or trusting of the love she was receiving from her partners. The very love she was seeking became a threat because it was unbelievable to a persona that was never good enough and thought of itself so poorly. Such a lonely way to live.

She had to see that the messages her mother gave her, in this case through neglect, were about her mother's deficits and inabilities to attend and nurture. *It was never about her.* The belief that she was not good enough was just not true, and never had been.

We all have so many layers of shame, hurt, anger, resentment, and trauma to work through. Under those layers and behind the programming and patches lie our most innocent and free essence that is naturally whole and unbroken. It is usually through our conditioned and constructed patchwork personas that we experience ourselves, others, circumstances, and the world around us in ways that ultimately hurt and isolate us. Once we begin to see through the eyes of our heart, the world and those in it change.

YOUR INNER CHILD IS INNOCENT

I was eating lunch with my ex-wife, who was pregnant with her first baby. I asked her if she could sense or feel the spirit or consciousness of her baby.

She paused and said, "I'm not sure, but I feel something."

"What is it like?" I asked.

And she responded, "Pure and soft."

I realized right then that this is what I am pointing clients toward in our PP work and what I know to be true of each and every one of us. Under the layers and patches lies something pure and soft. My ex-wife was speaking about our original essence.

Connect to that part of you that existed before the programming, before shame and self-criticism took hold of your consciousness and cast a shadow over your heart. Your heart is pure and unconditioned. Love your inner child, who needs your attention, tenderness, nurturance, encouragement, and support to live and play freely in the field of your soul, unbound by the opinions and judgments of others.

Remove those patches and let your raw, authentic self dance in the fresh spring rain.

After all, this is what we are all longing for—to be free and fully ourselves. Now let us learn how psychedelic psychotherapy can help us do just that.

CHAPTER 4

THE NEXT YOU
AUTHENTIC AND ALIGNED

Danny, a thirty-two-year-old firefighter, wanted to build his confidence. He was known as an excellent firefighter, loved by the people in his and other stations. He was dependable and worked hard. But inside, he was a mess.

He struggled with low self-esteem and was always on guard and near-panicked that his girlfriend would abruptly reject him and leave. A previous girlfriend had cheated on him, and it had ended the relationship, but his fear and paranoia were beyond reasonable and overwhelmed him most of the day, every day.

The fear was so bad he spent much of his days fighting himself not to text his girlfriend for reassurance. When he lost this inner battle, he would text her and share his anxieties, and she would respond saying she loved him and was happy in the relationship. He really wanted to believe her. He liked her so much. But ...

Her reassurances worked for a little while, but like a drug that wears off much too quickly, he found himself wanting to text her again with the same concerns. Her reassuring him unfortunately reinforced his desires to check in with her rather than enabling him to soothe and tend to himself, so the torturous cycle continued.

Well into his high school years, he had been the type of child who stayed and played by himself on the playground, always afraid of being embarrassed and ridiculed. He continued to live with these fears in adulthood and made himself into the image he perceived others wanted him to be: strong, funny, charming, bold, and courageous. But to him, this was a persona that would one day fall apart to reveal someone unsuitable, cowardly, not worth the effort.

He was tired of the obsessive nature of his mind and the overwhelming urges to find reassurance from others about his worth. Being extremely insightful, he knew he needed confidence in himself. He wanted to know he was good enough regardless of whether people stayed or left.

During one of our prep sessions, we practiced a future-oriented meditation where he saw himself the way he hoped to become: with good posture, making direct eye contact, laughing, being good-natured and friendly, feeling secure and comfortable with himself. At first, he couldn't recognize himself and distrusted his own imagination. But as the meditation continued, he saw that this was in fact him, just older and wiser and much more confident.

He sensed what it felt like to *feel* that way and brought some of the feeling into his body. Light as it was, he touched confidence and self-love and knew what to move toward in our work. He reflected later that this was what he had been looking for most of his life, and he felt a sense of hope for the first time in a very long time.

Thus began our journey toward self-love and confidence in who he really was.

In addressing the patchwork persona, we acknowledge some of what causes existential distress and exacerbates mental health issues such as depression and anxiety. So, how does psychedelic psychotherapy contribute to moving us from despair and distress to our desired change? We don't just want to heal; we also want to grow. But grow toward what?

Our future self, our next self.

Time and time again, I have witnessed how clients see and then dismantle the conditioning and programming that no longer serve them, including the values and beliefs instilled by parents, caretakers, teachers and preachers, and the dominant culture. Of course, not all values and beliefs are "wrong" for the client, but many were not chosen freely from within the space of one's own heart, which makes all the difference.

It's not that these conditioned beliefs are erased in psychedelic sessions but that clients become much more aware of them and how they are underlying unconscious drivers of their behaviors. Once aware, clients can then choose more freely what they want to believe based on who they are right then. After the sessions, they can choose to return to the old beliefs or keep forging ahead toward a future built on their own.

Moving toward "the next you" is the process of discovering the values, ethics, attitudes, and behaviors of your future selves and then practicing embodying this way of being *in the present*. Right now, if you start practicing how your ideal future self *is*, you literally become that version of yourself. If you do nothing right now, you will continue to be this version of yourself in the future. And there may be nothing "wrong" with that at all! For the most part, it's completely up to you who you want to be in the future. In one of his dharma talks, the influential Zen master Suzuki Roshi said it best: "Each of you is perfect the way you are . . . and you can use a little improvement."

So the question is, Are you the way you want to be?

I'd like to introduce you to a process I employ with clients to help them become their "next you." If we can imagine or visualize what our future self is doing and what it looks like, acts like, and feels like, we can begin to move in the direction of embodying that self now. Let's not leave our future up to chance or allow it to be dictated by the limiting conditions of our past. We have agency in what can unfold for ourselves.

If you long to be more present and peaceful, imagine your future self already *being* these ways. See how she is with herself and her friends; visualize how he is with his children and spouse. Clearly see them being present and at peace in their day. That is you in a potential future where you are being the way you long to be. Now, imagine feeling those ways in your body right now. Peaceful and calm, present and aware. Just for a moment, step into your future self.

You can start this process now! You don't need to wait to engage in psychedelic psychotherapy to practice these new ways of being. But, dang, it sure is hard to keep it up without support. And this is why this type of therapy is so helpful.

A PATH TO DISCOVERING YOUR INNATE GOODNESS

Put simply, during psychedelic psychotherapy, the client
- Becomes more aware of the conditioning and unconscious programming that run their life by investigating the feeling of being misaligned with who they really are in the context of their life.
- Applies compassion and love like a salve to the parts wounded by the way these values and beliefs were taught to them and how they affected them. (This could be considered inner child work: going back in time to witness themselves when they first felt confused or hurt by the messages they received and how they received them.)
- Discovers what Zen Buddhists would call their *original face* — their innate goodness, innocence, and purity. (Often

> this is when clients see how innocent they were as children before the shame set in.)
> - Discovers the truths, values, and beliefs that are unique to them beneath their conditioning and programming. (What is unique to them comes forward in session.)
> - Speaks these truths and commits to bringing them forward in their life by aligning their values, ethics, and beliefs with behaviors to create authenticity, confidence, and empowerment.

The problem is not that we don't want these changes but that these changes require us to make a significant shift in our self-perception. Our conditioning, programming, habits, and patterns are so strong, and we are ironically so attached to these old ways of being, that it takes dissolving the very ego that holds them so tightly to create the space and freedom to act in a new way, the way your future self is already being.

If you can imagine your future self living in alignment and being authentic, then you can begin to move in that direction. It's simple. But not easy. Let's take a closer look at what I mean by alignment.

ALIGNMENT

The more I do this work, the clearer it becomes that when people's lives are misaligned with their purpose and values, there is suffering. When their lives are aligned with their deepest truths and there is authenticity, there is thriving, resiliency, and joy.

Even when life becomes difficult, the people who are aligned and authentic face their challenges with confidence, trust, and courage, knowing they can depend on themselves, and they are also not afraid to ask for support to move through.

Psychedelic psychotherapy can help us align in the following ways:

- Align with our true identity and innocence
- Align with our core values
- Align with our inner wisdom and intuition
- Align with who we'd like to be
- Align with our body

Aligning with Our True Identity and Innocence

In Zen Buddhism, we are encouraged to reflect on what our "original face looked like before we were born." Though a strange prompt at first, it points directly to our identity being intimately connected to all the forces and influences of not only our ancestry but also the world itself.

We cannot pull our parents out of us (no matter how badly we may want to!). We also cannot pull sunlight, river water, cloud, rain, wind, dust and dirt, insects and animals, garbage and roses out of us. The same goes for our concept of "me," which is an amalgamation of ancestors, parents, caregivers, culture, and all human history.

Psychedelic experiences help people uncover the various layers of identity they tend to associate with or are attached to. And as these layers are uncovered and drop away, what remains, for many, is an ineffable sense of being that is unconditioned, pure, and formless. I've heard it described as boundless, infinite space, pure awareness, endlessly expansive, quiet and still. Its quality is most often compared to love.

As stated at the end of the previous chapter, our original nature is pure and innocent, unconditioned by beliefs, traumas, learning, information, and programming. This is what so many clients report while on the medicine and during therapy. They begin to see themselves the way they see babies and children. They also become much more aware of how they are treating themselves in their daily lives.

I cannot count how many times I've heard, "I would never treat anybody else the way I treat myself." I remember working with one of my clients, a deeply spiritual sixty-year-old window cleaner and former Christian pastor, on him talking to himself with kindness, support, and encouragement rather than self-hatred and deprecation. This was his most difficult task to date. As he went through ketamine treatment, he began to recognize his own innocence as a child, before he was shamed out of it by a stepparent and a teacher. He saw his innate, sweet, and playful self, which he said was beaten out of him at an early age. He saw himself being belittled as a young child, made to feel small and insignificant. He saw his shame and how that influenced so many behaviors and decisions he made in his life: how he was driven to control others; punish and deny himself; fall into a deep, existential despair. During these sessions, he connected to this innocence and felt it swell within him, leaving him feeling whole again.

During the later integration phase of therapy (detailed in Chapter 10), as he directed self-love and kindness toward himself, he noticed his mind returning to its old habit of being hateful. He would often talk in awe about his granddaughter, whom he loved more than anyone else besides his wife, so I asked if he would ever speak to her that way. "No way! It hurts to even think about that." Knowing he would actually never do it, I suggested that, until he was committed and firm in talking to himself with kindness, he should talk to his granddaughter the same way he talked to himself. He laughed, but I said seriously, "See what happens."

The next week, he reported that he couldn't bring himself to do it and so caught himself every time he started to berate or belittle himself. He asked himself, "Isn't my soul just as precious and deserving of love and kindness?" This was the major insight that he needed to commit to his new behaviors. This would stick.

He has since made a habit of catching himself in self-hating talk and choosing to be kind and supportive, rather than punishing and demanding, instead. Although the old habit still arises, it comes much less frequently and passes quickly. He has learned to cherish his own innocence and pure heart, which he no longer punishes.

In psychedelic psychotherapy, as in other psychedelic experiences, we have the opportunity to *feel* this purity and innocence. Self-loathing and self-hatred are usually learned in childhood. During a PP session, when a self-loathing client witnesses their younger self before all the learned negative beliefs and critical judgments set in and feels the love, true and lasting healing takes place. As I state throughout this book, unconditional love is the strongest medicine.

For me, there is nothing more beautiful than witnessing someone seeing their original nature, seeing their own innocence. So many weep when they discover the purity of their childhood self, and on many occasions this comes with the realization, "It wasn't my fault."

Seeing this (or knowing this already) during psychedelic psychotherapy brings immediate and immeasurable freedom, peace, and ease. Whereas the good *feelings* that come with this alignment and recognition do not last, the truth of what one *is* does. And like all truths, it needs to become a daily practice to remind ourselves of this truth often until we fully integrate and embody it.

Aligning with Our Core Values

Not only can we connect with our original face, but we can also (re)discover, develop, and align with our own set of values, beliefs, and ethics, which may not be those of our caretakers, parents, or culture.

People who grew up in a strictly religious context and who later choose to "leave the church" and establish their lives around values that better align with who they are demonstrate putting this type of alignment into action. Many who have left the church come to therapy having no sense of who they are under the layers of conditioning of their upbringing. As adults, they discover themselves for the first time, both a confusing and a liberating experience.

This is an obvious example of individuals whose core sense of self could be mired and bogged down beneath others' values, expectations, and beliefs. It is as true for those leaving the church as it is for the rest of us. An individual does not need to have been born and raised in a religious context to walk away from the dominant beliefs of their culture or upbringing. To be fair and clear, many of the values put forward by a religion or the dominant culture can be beneficial and good for the betterment of humanity and the world; we do not need to dismiss them out of hand or turn away from them all. The point is that our individual well-being depends on us *consciously* choosing and aligning with the values and beliefs that work for us personally.

> Four things can become clear during psychedelic psychotherapy:
>
> 1. From even before birth, but specifically afterward, we are programmed and conditioned to take on others' beliefs, values, and worldviews that have nothing to do with us personally.
> 2. We may or may not be aligned with, and want to stay committed to, those values, beliefs, ethics, and worldviews.
> 3. There may be grief, anger, resentment, confusion, fear, and relief in seeing this discrepancy clearly.
> 4. Listening to one's own heart often reveals inherent core values and that which often lies hidden, repressed, denied, or dormant.

What is most important to healing and growth is that people have the awareness and agency to *consciously choose* what is right for them at that time in their lives. This is alignment, and it helps create the best conditions in which greater mental health and well-being can arise and be sustained.

Aligning with Our Intuition and Wisdom

One of the most potent forms of alignment is learning to hear, and *listen to*, our inner voice, which we find not in our head but in our gut and heart. This is not metaphorical but literal—the voice of intuition and wisdom is often heard *coming from* those places in the body. It's a voice arising from the deep, with qualities of doubtless calm knowing.

This is our intuition and our wisdom speaking.

How many times have you heard but dismissed or even denied this voice?

I certainly have, and more times than I care to admit.

I distinctly remember hearing that voice one time. "Don't do it, Mikey. That's going to cause a lot of trouble." And yet I did it anyway, and it caused me, and others, a lot of trouble and hurt.

Although intuition and wisdom are different—one arises from our senses and the other from lived experience—they both offer invaluable information, especially when we face important decisions. Yet, in the West especially, we are conditioned to *not* pay attention to these deeper forms of knowing, often at our own expense and peril.

The cognitive, intellectual mind holds information, but it cannot make up its own mind. This mind plays Ping-Pong with itself—this, that, yes, no, maybe, I don't know, what she said, what he wants . . . on and on. And this is what we've been trained to listen to while making decisions. No wonder we are often paralyzed by choice and confused.

Psychedelic psychotherapy, like certain meditation practices, helps bring clarity and discernment. We can hear and listen to our intuition and our inner wisdom, that found in our body, in our heart.

So many of my clients report hearing and then forming a relationship with their inner voice. It guides them, after sessions, toward healthier decisions and more skillful behaviors.

Aligning with Our Future

> *Until one is committed, there is hesitancy, the chance to draw back, always ineffectiveness. Concerning all acts of initiative (and creation), there is one elementary truth, the ignorance of which kills countless ideas and splendid plans: that the moment one definitely commits oneself, then Providence moves too. All sorts of things occur to help one that would never otherwise*

have occurred. A whole stream of events issues from the decision, raising in one's favour all manner of unforeseen incidents and meetings and material assistance, which no man could have dreamt would have come his way. I have learned a deep respect for one of Goethe's couplets:

*Whatever you can do, or dream you can, begin it.
Boldness has genius, power, and magic in it. Begin it now!*
—William Hutchinson Murray, "Until One Is Committed"

Infinite potential futures are ready to greet you. One small decision you make today can create a trajectory that could change your life completely in the future. Thus, your future is open and remains a mystery. Although we have virtually no control over external forces that act on us and force decisions, we do retain agency and have the ability to influence *who we are* in our future.

What is almost guaranteed is, if you do not make conscious changes, your future is likely to follow the same pattern as your past (barring external circumstances).

Who is the one making decisions for you? The patchwork persona who moves to the expectations and dictates of others, or your unconditioned heart that moves to its own rhythm, finding a way forward of its own accord? The future you are longing or hoping for is possible (reasonably so, of course!). If you can *imagine* a future version of yourself that is thriving, aligned, and authentic, you can start to *become* it. (To be clear, I am speaking of the quality of your future life, not necessarily what you will be doing in it. This is not a future wish list or fantasy list but rather who you want to be.)

In psychedelic psychotherapy, seeing and imagining a future different from the past becomes possible and easier as the ego's defensive, constricting limits on our consciousness begin to release and our consciousness expands. It can be difficult for the mind in a present state of depression or anxiety to imagine anything different. It's not depression or anxiety that is keeping one down or behind but actually the mind's attachment to those states.

I know, that's hard to believe at first.

But during psychedelic psychotherapy, it becomes clear how those very states arise to protect us from taking risks and chances, from putting ourselves first, from disobeying the conditions that were imposed on us.

When there is space outside the constricting limits we continue to place on ourselves, the mind is free, with the heart, to imagine new scenes, vistas, adventures, lifestyles, relationships, careers, and so on.

In a practice my colleague Cassandra Vieten and I call "futuremaking," the vibrant future self comes into being in imagination and leads us onward toward itself. One small change after another, we choose new behaviors and ways of being and begin to align with that vision.

During psychedelic psychotherapy, clients have the freedom to imagine new ways of being, to see a future self that is possible but that was not accessible before. Clients have seen versions of themselves that were patient, firm but kind, boundaried and protective of their own well-being, strong and empowered . . . this amazing list goes on and on. In session, they learn to have a relationship with this future self. When they ask the future self questions, it responds in a way that guides the client onward. They are accessing their innate wisdom that comes through the voice and presence of this imagined future self. When clients interact with their wiser, more empowered future self, it encourages them to set boundaries or to ask for what they need or to take whichever first steps will lead to that future state.

When the future self presents itself in session, the first prompt I give clients is to simply acknowledge it, say hello, and see if it has anything to share. Then, notice what it looks like, feels like, what it is doing. Some other prompts are as follows:

"How did you get there?"
"How can I become you?"
"How can I deal with this problem?"

Clients are not only accessing their inner wisdom but also creating a relationship with an *idea* of themselves that comes from beyond their conditioning. Though becoming this new version in one session is not possible because of the limits of current conditioning (neurological and psychological), the brain's neuroplasticity will allow this new version of self to be incorporated into daily life and practiced.

WWFSD? (What Would Future Self Do?)

Once a future self presents itself, a client has a new resource to rely on in difficult moments and for decision-making. Clients learn to access and speak to a future self in session, and I encourage them to practice communicating regularly. They can call on the future self to help choose a path that leads to that future version. To get to a place in the future that is different from where we are now calls for a new direction to be established with new behaviors. An imagined future self, making new decisions and healthier choices, acts as a model and can provide guidance on how to get there.

MEDITATION AND REFLECTION

You don't have to try psychedelic psychotherapy to discover this future version of yourself. You can try it now at **michaelsapiro.com /meditations**.

If you don't have access right now, then just close your eyes, take three slow, deep breaths, and settle into your body. In the space behind your eyes, imagine a version of yourself who is older. Without any limits, imagine your future self is engaged in doing something you've always wanted to do, living a life you've dreamed of. Where are you, and what are you doing in this vision? What are you wearing? What do your hair and facial features look like? How is your health? Imagine your future self turning to you and giving you advice about how to get to that place in the future. What do you say to yourself?

If you have a journal, this is a good time to reflect and take notes on the experience. What was it like for you? What was difficult? Could you see yourself in the future? Or just a form without details? Did you hear yourself and what did you say to you?

If you can see something, it is more likely to become a reality. If you can see yourself acting, thinking, speaking in new ways that are more aligned with your core values and authentic, then that self can become your reality.

A healthier, joyful, calm, peaceful, thriving, energized, and passionate future is waiting to be seen so it can be lived.

Start it now.

Aligning with Our Body

The body keeps the score. This phrase has been popularized by Bessel van der Kolk with his book of the same name, which discusses how trauma affects and changes the body and brain. I have seen myriad effects on the body: It is where difficult feelings are experienced, so of course so many of us have turned away from our body. But our body is also where we feel joy, love, and peace. To turn away from one set of feelings is to shut ourselves off from the other. The emotions my clients are hoping to experience cannot be felt in isolation; they arise with other emotions. So, to be a fully embodied person who *feels* life as it is lived, one has to live *in* the body.

Imagine playing your favorite song but keeping the volume down so low you can barely hear it. What would that be like? Dull and frustrating! Tuning out your body is like this—life feels flat. To live the life you want, aligning with your body is essential. That means paying attention to emotions, sensations, energy, pains, and pleasures.

> *The good news:* No matter how long you've numbed yourself to your body, you can realign and connect to it almost immediately.
> *The bad news:* You have to feel your feelings in this process.
> *The good news:* You can now feel life's vibrancy within and around you: Colors are brighter, sounds are clearer, foods taste better, joy is felt, and even ecstasy can become a regular expression of life. All are felt in the body.
> *The bad news:* Why are you always looking for the bad news?!

The body not only feels and senses but also contains wisdom that is accessible when we learn to listen to its signals—gut feelings, hunches, constrictive warnings, goosebumps of wonder and awe, Spidey senses, basically. Gavin de Becker's *The Gift of Fear* clearly details how our intuition and ability to sense our environment (including other people's intentions) are our primary defenses against danger. He suggests that most victims of violence sensed the danger before it occurred, but they were not trained to *believe* what they *felt*.

In general, our body constricts and tightens when something is not right and expands and relaxes when in alignment with what is right or true. You can demonstrate this for yourself right now. Take a moment to think of a circumstance that was challenging for you, then notice your body's response. Now take a moment to think about an experience when you felt at home, at ease. What is your body's response? When you need to make an important decision and your mind is a tennis match between ideas, between yeses and noes, take a moment to tune in to your body. Right now, think of a decision you want to make. Sit with the decision. Imagine saying yes. What is your body's response? Imagine saying no. What is your body's response?

When we attune to and align with our body, we not only gain access to our innate wisdom but also receive information from the surrounding world. There is so much information in the body and in how it responds to stimuli and circumstance. Through our body, we attune to our environment. During medicine work and after, our senses are opened and heightened, able to tap into the hidden matrix of infinite data that exists beneath our usually dulled senses.

Waking up the senses is waking up to life.

There is not one dull moment in life, only a dulled mind and numbed-out body.

It is no surprise that so many good books and training programs incorporate the body into treatment of mental health issues. Generally, this is not a focus in most therapy programs, but the field is now much more aware of the importance of tuning in to the body for optimal overall health. Yogis have known this for millennia. And so have many traditional medicine practices that we are only now beginning to understand through advanced science techniques and technological advances.

We are not floating heads living in a meat suit. We are and our consciousness is housed in a living, feeling, sensing conscious ecosystem. When we learn to pay attention to our body, our life expands to include what's vast in and around us. If you can feel an angry person as they enter the room, imagine what it would *feel* like to encounter a mountain range or the trees in a thick forest in the same way.

Psychedelic psychotherapy wakes us up, makes us more aware, and helps us see the body as vital to life, not just a place we live and can ignore or abuse. Our well-being and ability to thrive in the future depend on our relationship with our body, where life is felt and experienced. We want to go from living life in an isolated, contained thought bubble to feeling the vibrancy of life in the present moment. This starts in the body with our awareness of our senses and feelings.

AUTHENTICITY

When you think of people who are authentic, who comes to mind? What are their traits and characteristics? Are they characters—dress funky, dance with wild abandon, speak their minds, and share their hearts? Do they march to the beat of their own drum and create their own culture and customs to live by? What makes them authentic?

Two common statements I hear from new clients are "I just want to be myself" and "I don't really know who I am." These sentiments are often paired with anxiety and depression, but instead of focusing on the symptoms, in therapy we focus on what is authentic in them and how to bring that forward in their lives for greater alignment. Those two statements are not just superfluous data points but important gates that lead clients down a path toward their original nature and who they really are beneath all the conditioning.

The COVID-time experience made it surprisingly clear that so many people were unfulfilled by their careers and relationships. Clients who came to me both before and after COVID had different ideas of what growth meant to them and what they wanted for themselves. Doug's story is a good example: COVID ruined Doug's business. The stresses of dealing with the regulations and rules and the distancing were hard enough, but when he couldn't pay the rent, he knew he had to close the doors. His whole identity was wrapped up in being a business owner and accountant. Though he was never really a drinker, he started using in the evenings, which turned into day drinking.

Though he had been pushed into earning a business degree by his father, who was a banker, and he later fell into being an accountant, Doug felt a sense of pride in owning his own business. Yet he always felt a deep longing to do what he had dreamed of doing when he was younger, but he knew he was living up to his father's expectations. When his business closed, he fell into despair; he felt ashamed and like a failure.

But something in him woke up and he sought help. He couldn't motivate himself to go back to accounting and felt stuck. In our first prep session, I asked him what the longing was that he'd mentioned. He said it was a silly idea, which was a clue that he felt really connected to it, so I started pulling on that thread.

As a child, he and his mother would watch baking shows together on Saturday mornings, then practice making the recipes in the afternoons. Think flour everywhere, laughter, wonderful smells of home-baked goods, and warmth. He felt safe and happy. Then his mother became sick with cancer and died when he was fifteen.

It was then Doug decided to become a baker, not only to honor his mother but also because he was truly happy in the kitchen baking. While his friends engaged in sports, he worked at local bakeries. While his friends bought the latest video games, he bought ingredients. Unfortunately, his father did not support this dream and would not pay for culinary school. If Doug wanted college paid for, he had to study business, which he did. And the baking dream died.

During his first ketamine session, he returned to the kitchen and saw his mother again. His grief, still alive and in his body, flooded out and he wept. He could smell the cakes, feel her presence. She looked at him and said, "Do what you want to do, honey, this is your life." In the following session, he processed his feelings toward his father, for whom he felt respect and gratitude; nonetheless, he didn't feel seen or understood by the man. Doug was able to express the pain of having his dreams invalidated, and he started to feel a sense of connection to what was always there, but denied.

During our final ketamine session, he allowed himself to dream again. He saw a bakery, a logo, various pastries and cakes. He glowed a warmth that I could feel sitting next to him.

Fast-forward a year, and I receive a text with a photo of a storefront and a smiling Doug holding a cake. Although I cannot disclose the name of his bakery, I can attest it's legit, and his goods are delicious and full of love.

To generalize some of what I saw:

Pre-COVID clients seemed driven to succeed and accomplish, to do and to have more.

Post-COVID clients seem to be driven toward purpose and living meaningful lives, not wasting their precious life energy and time. I saw a shift toward spending more meaningful time with family and friends and working in an environment that was better suited to them.

I saw a shift from achievement to authenticity.

There is nothing wrong with ambition and achievement, but if the drive to succeed comes from a conditioned striving to be loved or to find one's worth, then the search tends to be never-ending, depressing, and exhausting.

Life is so different when we create our goals from a place of alignment and for the sake of being authentic. Then our self-worth does not depend on the success or failure of the goal. Rather, it is born out of how we support and encourage ourselves to reach our goals and see failures as learning opportunities.

Please know this is no small shift in perception or in the relationship we have with ourselves. The best conditions for sustaining embodied self-worth and self-love are created internally. And as discussed in the following chapters, psychedelic psychotherapy is a powerful method for cultivating this pivotal shift in mind and heart.

The psychedelic medicine helps reveal our defenses and patchwork personas, and at times it even helps dissolve them so that, as when clouds disperse and expose the sun, our innate goodness, wisdom, truth, and authenticity shine brightly. Truly being you, as weird as you may be, is exactly what it takes to be you.

During psychedelic psychotherapy, we learn to honor ourselves just as we are. The process encourages us to grow into the next healthier, more peaceful, energized, creative version of ourselves by living up to our potential and sharing this with our families, communities, and others across the globe. Your future self is waiting to be seen by you.

Let's now turn our attention to the process of psychedelic psychotherapy: from the preparation stages through the sessions into integration and finally toward living deeply.

PART TWO

THE WOUNDED HEART GOES ON A JOURNEY

Misty Mountains and Mud

His feet were bound
by chains or weight,
each step up
the forested slope,
a major force of will.

The pathway had grown over:
loose rocks, slugs, sharp shells,
broken branches, white bones,
slick dark mud under foot he felt.

His pace slow and labored,
he noticed more moving
at this painful, primal rhythm.

There were indentations in the mud
of footprints.
Short shuffled steps,
like his own,
leading up the path.

There were indentations in mud
of knees,
where others had fallen,
perhaps in prayer
or exhaustion.

There were indentations in mud
of foreheads,
splayed bodies,
where others had lain
posed prostrate in surrender.

Down in the mud, life was bustling:
ants marching,
chirping crickets jumping
from grass to rocks.

The sounds of birds,
the whoosh of wings,
from overhead he heard.

Sunlight
Wind
The soft babbling of a stream

CHAPTER 5

PREPARATION

DISCOVERING THE HEART
OF THE HURT

Grace, a woman in her early sixties, was a retired Army intelligence officer. She had spent the majority of her military career in intelligence, spending years gathering intelligence, training others to do the same, and analyzing people and organizations to predict and prevent acts of terror. What she knew about evil in the world never left her consciousness, and daily concerns of personal safety directed her behavior and invaded her dreams. She was never "off duty." She had rescued people during a military coup, protected confidential information, worked with multiple intelligence agencies to prevent an attack on National Guard troops on a peacekeeping mission—things out of a movie, only they happened in real time to a real person.

On one mission, while a multiagency effort was ongoing to prevent an attack on an embassy, she was given a DIP mission, or a die-in-place mission. If the combatants stormed her location, she was ordered to destroy highly confidential documents by pulling the pins on the grenades attached to the safe. What she remembers most about that situation was that the sergeant working under her did not seem to understand their orders and what would happen after they pulled the pins on the grenades. They had no real escape. The building and property were enclosed by high walls and barbed wire and broken glass on top of the walls. She remembered his confusion, but he was a good follower and obeyed orders. This was her duty, which she would fulfill without hesitation.

When reflecting on the incident, she was angry at the thought of how expendable she and that sergeant were to the military. She had wanted to be a mother, a schoolteacher, a member of a community, to live in safety, and she would have lost all that to possibly stop a terrorist organization, one that is still active today, from accessing information. For twenty-six years, her identity as a warrior and patriot dominated her consciousness. Now, more than thirty years after this particular event and more than a decade after military retirement, she still struggled to know who she really was.

Her father had been an officer in the Air Force, and like him, she had dedicated her life to her country and the missions of the US Armed Forces. But how about now? Even retired, she put her needs and her life aside for her mother, her sick brother, nonprofit organizations, and the various nonprofit boards of directors she served on. She continued to give herself away to greater missions. Now, retired, living in safety in a vibrant community, she was still plagued with concerns for safety and by horrific nightmares.

I asked Grace if caring for herself landed on her task list at all. She said it was so far down the list, she barely existed. She hadn't felt joy for years; she neglected playing music, which was a passion; she didn't really feel alive or interested in living at times. Through the prep sessions and into the ketamine treatment, it became clearer that she had been trained to neglect and deny herself. Her service was paired with martyrdom, and this was slowly killing her.

Saying no was not an option, or so it seemed. *Give until you die, till there is no more left of you.*

But her soul spoke loud enough for her to hear and brought her to me.

Regardless of the medicine or whether I am working with an individual, a group, or a retreat, preparation is one of the most essential tasks in all psychedelic therapies, especially in psychedelic psychotherapy. Preparation serves multiple purposes, and its importance for preparing both therapist and client to engage in this type of transformational work cannot be overstated. From my perspective, simply dropping into a therapeutic psychedelic experience without the necessary preparation can be unethical, confusing, and even harmful.

Preparation sets the stage for the work. It's when the therapist discusses potential risks and benefits and, through the informed consent process, makes sure the client knows what they are agreeing to. I use this time to discover the heart of the hurt, what needs healing, and where the edges of growth are. Preparation helps us orient toward what the client wants most out of the experience and in their life. While the medicine does what the medicine will, it is both the therapist's and the client's responsibility to uncover what is most seeking to be healed and what growth is most desired. Otherwise, a psychedelic session is like going into Trader Joe's without a shopping list—just not a good idea. It's like one of my patients saying, "I asked God for a change in my life, and then my wife left me! That was not what I meant!" Often, our intentions are unrealistic, unreasonable, or simply unclear. We need to be clear. We want to work in collaboration with life, so being clear about our intentions and therapeutic goals helps us get what we are actually longing for. In this chapter, I describe the informed consent process, working with expectations, how to prepare for the actual session, how to deal with the possibility of an ego death, and how to help clarify intentions.

A client and I may have as few as one or two prep sessions to get through all the necessary steps before we engage in therapy, so I have trained myself to be thorough in this preparation process while maintaining the love and compassion necessary to create a healthy therapeutic relationship. Doing thorough prep work leaves more room to focus on healing and growth during the sessions. I find the best outcomes happen when we have more time to prepare, so I ask my clients to schedule four to eight prep sessions, if possible, over one to two months. This is the ideal setup to ensure the greatest success.

INITIAL PREP SESSIONS

Before I meet with a client for our prep sessions, we have a short phone consultation to assess whether we are a good fit and to evaluate which medicine might be best for meeting their growth and healing goals. If they then pass their medical and psych screening, and we have determined we are a good therapeutic fit, then we set our first prep session.

The prep process differs depending on whether I am working with someone at the ketamine clinic, working with a private client, or leading an international retreat.

Ketamine Clinic Process
- Initial consult and medical or psych screening with the clinic director.
- Initial consultation with me to determine good therapeutic fit. (Am I the best therapist to work with them or might another therapist or healer be more appropriate?)
- Hour-long preparation call to discover the heart of the hurt, set intentions, talk about the psychedelic experience, and complete the informed consent process.
- I assign readings, podcasts, and journal activities.

- We meet for our first ketamine-assisted psychotherapy (KAP) session.

Process for Other Medicine Psychotherapies for Private Clients
- Initial call to assess for good fit, to hear the client's goals, and to choose the most appropriate medicine.
- Medical and psych screening call with a psychedelic-trained psych nurse or clinical psychedelic pharmacologist.
- Prep call or calls to discover the heart of the hurt, set intentions, talk about the psychedelic experience, and complete the informed consent process.
- I assign readings, podcasts, and journal activities.
- We meet for our first psychedelic psychotherapy session.

Retreat Process
- Clients are referred to the organization I work with by word of mouth, by their therapists, or through other organizations.
- They are screened by the psych nurse.
- They work with coaches to set intentions and prepare for the retreat.
- I meet with all the staff and participants to set the stage for the retreat, to meet and greet, to answer questions.
- I assign them extra readings, podcasts, meditations, and journal activities.
- We gather for the retreat.

INFORMED CONSENT AND THE THERAPEUTIC RELATIONSHIP

The informed consent process is essentially a mutually protective contract between the healer, therapist, or clinician and the client. It is there first and foremost so the client is fully aware of the risks and benefits of the therapy and has agency in deciding what works or does not work for them before they begin the transformational journey. The process gives the therapist a chance to share what the client can expect from them and the process and to set appropriate and healthy boundaries. During the informed consent process, the client is made aware of the potential medical risks of the therapy and is asked to make a collaborative plan in case an emergency arises during session.

An informed consent document may discuss the following topics:

- Potential risks and benefits of engaging in psychedelic psychotherapy, including adverse reactions to the medicine and any psychological distress that may arise
- Limits of confidentiality based on state laws and what is disclosed during the session (Yep, if a client shares anything in session that falls under mandated reporting law, even while under the influence of the medicine, it is reportable.)
- The potential use of therapeutic touch and the client's right to revoke this consent anytime in the process
- Boundaries around sexually explicit or aggressive behaviors
- Detailed emergency procedures
- Cancellation policy

The informed consent process allows the client to have a voice in their treatment and healing process. "Yes, I agree to these terms" is an essential part of the preparation and therapeutic process. Having a say and agency in one's own treatment is essential, and too many people have already been stripped of this agency by others and harmful institutional medical practices. The consent process itself is empowering. A good informed consent process creates the right conditions for the work to unfold safely for the client. Trust is established between the client and the healer when clients know up front that their well-being is the most important factor in the work.

FOR THERAPISTS

To engage in psychedelic psychotherapy is a courageous act for a client, and to trust a therapist requires even more courage. Relationship building is an essential part of the prep process. The therapist must know what a sacred honor it is to work with people in expanded states of consciousness and how brave someone who is suffering is to entrust themselves to the care of a stranger. In fact, the bravery and courage to trust another may be mediating factors in psychedelic psychotherapy.

I cannot overstate what an honor and responsibility it is to sit with, guide, and do therapy with people in this state. I strongly believe that all therapists must have integrity and strong ethics to participate in this line of work. I encourage all my students to read *The Ethics of Caring* by Kylea Taylor to prepare themselves for this work. Everyone involved in this process has prep work to do, not just the clients.

DISTINGUISHING THE NORTH STAR FROM FALSE STARS: INTENTION SETTING

Setting intentions is one of the most important parts of the journey. It provides space for the heart to make itself known. How often do we depress what is most important to us, hide, bury, or guard it behind defensive walls or under layers of shame, guilt, self-criticism, numbness, resentment and anger, despair and grief? Setting intentions is a process of giving attention to what we long for. We do this by saying it out loud and having it witnessed by another.

Remember, taking this journey is not about what we don't want but rather about what we do want. One veteran on a retreat stated, "I just don't want to be angry anymore. It's fucking up my relationship to my kids." When I asked what he wanted, he wasn't sure. Then I asked him to take a moment to drop into his heart space and feel out his intentions. After a pause, he said, "I want to feel at peace." But I probed deeper: "For what purpose do you want to be at peace?" And without hesitation he replied, "I want to be more present with myself and my family. I want them to feel peace around me, for me to feel peace inside myself so I am easier to be around." This is a much clearer intention. In session, we then could target the reasons he was not at peace and enable him to actually feel that peace in real time, not only during the session but also in his daily life afterward.

A woman in her forties wanted to work with me after she'd left the corporate world and separated from her husband of many years. She was struggling with depression and self-worth issues. In the first prep session, we went right to her personas and where they were formed in her life. Here is her reflective email from the following day where she explores some of the patches that created a variety of her personas:

> Good to meet yesterday. I came away with a lot of reflection points. After sitting for a moment to catch my breath from the internal tsunami, several characters or personas came into clear focus—in addition to Corporate White Dude (CWD), who was the main character driving most of my 30s. It also became evident what needs each of these characters fulfills.
> The prospect of letting go of certain characters is terrifying because this removes the illusion of control in my life. CWD guided me toward success on the material plane, even if my heart was left unfulfilled. To some degree, I'm grateful for this service. External achievement has been comfortable. It's predictable and familiar, if not

sustainable—or desirable—in the long run. The disdain I feel at the prospect of being mediocre is a huge deterrent in being able to move forward, in trust, into the unknown.

Either way, now there's no way back. CWD's glory days are over. This strategy isn't working anymore. So I can continue to languish in misery, buoyed by excuses as to why my life fell apart, or dare to try something new. Even writing the latter feels uncomfortable. What would new feel like? Look like? Taste like? How would it feel to be enough right now, already, as you mentioned yesterday? I have no idea. But I'm keen to move ahead with this work to begin uncovering some of these answers.

She displayed such clarity in knowing what she no longer wanted to feel and what drove those parts of her to create a lifestyle and mindset she didn't want. Our next session was aimed at discovering what needed healing and what she wanted to move toward in our work.

THE FOUR DOMAINS AND OTHER PRACTICES

To facilitate the process of clarifying intentions, I've developed an activity I call "The Four Domains," in which I ask clients to reflect on what needs healing and what growth they are seeking.

The four domains are *physiological, psychological, spiritual,* and *ancestral*. Although we could start with so many other domains and prompts, I have found the most successful therapeutic outcomes occur when clients reflect on their hopes for healing and growth in these four specific domains. We are all looking for healing and growth, but we rarely specify what needs healing and where the growth should be, and these four domains cover so much ground. The following descriptions are not exhaustive.

Physiological Domain

Clients come in with chronic pain, headaches, cancer diagnoses, and the normal aches and pains of living in a body that is aging. The domain of the body, the physiological domain, includes diseases, discomforts, disorders, pain, how we take care of our body, and how we treat our body. I ask clients to think of their relationship with the various systems of the body, including the cardiovascular, pulmonary, endocrine, immune, neurological, and reproductive systems, and to reflect on the skin, bones, blood, hair, organs, heart, nails, eyes, and other body parts. Many clients have eating disorders, substance and alcohol abuse issues, body image issues, chronic fatigue, burnout and stress, and so many more presentations of a body hurting or not well taken care of.

Clients want to talk about eating, drinking, smoking, exercise, sex and sensuality, and drug use. In our prep sessions, I might ask them to reflect on the foods, drugs, alcohol, nicotine, coffee, sugars, meats, plants, and fruits they consume and whether they want to change any of these habits. I'm interested in better understanding what started their habits and when. We begin to focus on what happened in their life when they formed a harmful relationship with their body, food, or substances. I am not as interested in helping them change their habits as I am in healing what caused those habits in the first place. Those who address the deeper issues while learning to love their body succeed in making the long-lasting changes they desire. It's not the cigarette that's the issue; it's the compulsive need for soothing or stimulation.

Psychological Domain

Clients come in to address a range of mental and emotional concerns and issues, including core and limiting beliefs, attachment styles, thought patterns, self-talk habits, social and intimate relationship needs, emotional tolerance or dysregulation, communication skills, ego defenses and strengths, behaviors, presenting disorders like anxiety and depression, and trauma history.

In the psychological domain, clients usually begin to identify harmful beliefs about themselves, others, or the world writ large that *create* their reality. If after a significant trauma we believe the world is a dangerous place (and it certainly can be), we use that lens when out in the world and see everything interpreted through that belief. Vigilance can keep us safe, but hypervigilance locks us in a perpetual state of fear and stress, dysregulating the nervous system and polluting the body with chronic output of adrenaline and cortisol, which leads to a number of complicated health issues.

In a prep session, we may address how the client's attachment style, formed early in life with their primary caregiver, affects the way they operate in relationships in the present. Some struggle to lean in during challenges and prefer to run; others do not know how to create healthy boundaries and hold tightly when it is best to let go.

As I will state over and over again, we can prep and identify what clients most want to address, but during the therapeutic sessions, the medicine does what the medicine will. We must remain open to where the heart leads during psychedelic sessions. That said, doing deep and thorough prep work is as important as the medicine day itself. Once hidden or deeper issues are revealed, a client has a target, whether for medicine day or for later when they feel ready to address it.

Spiritual Domain

Clients bring in a wide range of religious and spiritual beliefs that influence their lives in ways we can address in prep and therapeutic sessions. Some clients who have been traumatized by religious institutions and systems purposefully do not think about spirituality; yet, when I ask about this particular domain directly, many state they are open to exploring this part of themselves. Some of the topics that arise include the meaning and purpose of life, a sense of belonging to the whole, and connection to one's self, others, the world, God, the universe, the divine, the earth, plants and animals, and so forth.

Spirituality can include daily practices such as meditation, deep breathing, dancing, drumming, prayer, and contemplation and rituals to honor the elements, ancestors, those who are sick, and those in need of support. Many aging clients and those dealing with cancer diagnoses come ready to create a healthy and positive relationship with death and reflect on their beliefs about life after death.

Ancestral Domain

Ancestral trauma and inherited trauma, although fairly new topics in therapy, are also common themes my clients bring to the table. Addressing the ancestral domain may include completing a cultural genogram to better understand the trials and tribulations, gifts and strengths, traumas and resiliency of our ancestors. What has been passed down and how does it influence and affect our thought patterns, behaviors, and decision-making? This domain covers ancestors' religion, spiritual beliefs, rituals and practices, how they made meaning in their lives, eating habits, substance use, specific historical and cultural traumas and events, gifts and passions, strengths and resiliencies, and beliefs around working, money, relationships, and the like.

Through the science of epigenetics, we are learning how ancestry, intergenerational trauma, and historical events influence our biology, thinking patterns, and behaviors. My clients are often surprised when they research, as best they can, the influence of their ancestors on their own lives. Doing so gives them surprising and important pieces of their puzzle that were unclear before.

The Four Domains exercise helps clients identify and discern their growth and healing intentions, which might at first not be obvious or drawn out. Along with this specific practice, I give clients reflection and writing exercises to help them prepare and keep their

THE FOUR DOMAINS EXERCISE

I would like to offer you an opportunity to try the Four Domains exercise because it can be a powerful reminder of what needs to be seen, expressed, and given your attention.

INSTRUCTIONS

- On a big piece of paper, please draw a large circle and divide it into four quarters. Write the names of the four domains at the top of each quarter.
- Choose one domain and set a timer for five minutes. During the five minutes, please respond to this prompt: In the following domain, what needs healing and what growth are you wanting?
- Spend time reflecting on where you are stuck, what needs attention, what needs to change, and what you feel about each. You can write or draw any symbols, signs, or images associated with the domain.
- When the time is up, set the timer for another five minutes and go through the process with the next domain. Complete the circle, addressing each of the four domains.

Once you complete this activity, spend a few moments reflecting on how you feel and what new insights arose.

---

mind focused. I want them to spend time reflecting and paying close attention to what they've chosen to focus on in our work, such as when they dwell in drama, indulge in self-pity, slide down the shame spiral, or listen to and believe overly critical thinking.

I ask them to keep a journal of thoughts, behaviors, urges, and impulses to build their self-awareness of what is actually going on inside them, where their suffering is the strongest. I also ask them to begin practicing the self-compassion and love they yearn for as soon as they witness self-judgment and then to write about the experience in their journal.

But sometimes, I have to get creative with the preparation exercises.

REDISCOVERING JOY

I was working with a world-class musician and producer who came to me for help addressing his chronic exhaustion and lack of joy. He'd begun playing the drums at three years old, under his father's tutelage, and it did not take long for "playing" to become "training." Under the guidance of a very particular, rigid, and detail-oriented father, who was a gigging musician himself, my client grew up associating perfection with self-worth. He also learned that, to earn his father's respect and love, he was not to miss a beat, literally.

He shared that he no longer was having fun in his career, struggled in his relationship, and was chronically exhausted, which he attributed to the stresses of touring and the constant demands in the recording studio. Even though he had played thousands of gigs, he would almost panic before each show, imagining he would not know how to play. He could relax only when on his seat and the show began, which was the only time he found his flow.

After following the thread of these feelings and beliefs, it became clear to us both that his exhaustion and depression were existential. Life, it seemed to him, was work. Making music, work. Making love, work.

If he didn't execute flawlessly, he failed.

If he wasn't perfect in his performance, he was a failure.

That *is* tiring. Living up to unrealistic expectations is exhausting because we can't ever get there and we literally destroy ourselves trying. I know this personally.

The musician and I met for our first prep session and agreed to work together. In the second prep session, we talked about his yearning to be free, to be spontaneous, to feel joy and ease.

To address how attached he was to "being perfect"—it was, after all, how he earned his father's love—he needed to see how trapped he truly was by these conditions and beliefs. Once he saw it, he could then blow up his self-made prison and set his heart free. And this is when I heard a song and thought of a plan for the next few preparation sessions.

Because of its strong emotionality, I had him listen to Renaud Garcia-Fons and Clair Antonini's "Nove alla Turca" and encouraged him to relax into the music as if he were getting into a warm bath. I asked him to witness his experience and write it down after.

His experience with the song suggests a mind overworking, a mind unwilling to relax its hold on his consciousness. He texted me his thoughts afterward:

> I tried to keep coming back to the experience of feeling it. Let it wash over me.
>
> Let me describe some thoughts that I had on the first listen, even when trying to just let it wash over me. Thinking about the piece, the choices in form and construction, influences, playing, instruments, their technique, cultural stylistic musical language mishmash, the mix panning choices, the bass overdub... wait... yup, that's an overdub, mix level rides, the stereo recording of the guitar or lute (not sure—lots of thinking on that), pretty sure that's an upright, but, man, does he play really high and in tune, is it a cello, no can't be, would I like it better if the lute instrument was recorded mono instead of with two mics and had a simpler seat in the stereo field, do I generally like that? How are they getting that bass tone, that reverb, does it contribute to the octave overtone that pokes out in certain bass notes...

He wasn't able to disconnect, to just let the music wash over him. We debriefed this in the context of his childhood conditioning, the effects of chronic perfectionism on his personality, and the cost of having to be extremely detailed oriented. He reported that he struggled to finish projects because there was always something to work on. His heart yearned to spend time with his wife, to dance more, to be playful. But his reality was bogged down in details and proving himself—these were his persona patches.

Again, I wanted him to just feel the music rather than analyze it, so I assigned Calle Rasmusson's beautiful "October" and encouraged him to listen with his heart and body, to be aware of emotions, sensations, memories, and images. Here is his response:

> This one was great, I was able to sync into it.
>
> Was helpful what you wrote, about feeling, images, memories, the heart.
>
> First assignment, when I had critical thoughts about the music, I tried to come back to the music and not think those thoughts. But listening to music is linked to those thoughts. Heavily reinforced.
>
> The second time I didn't just try to not think critical thoughts, I had a new focus to replace the old one. Watch and feel internally for images, feelings, etc.
>
> When I want my dogs to stop doing something, just telling them to stop works only momentarily if they have a lot of drive to do the thing they're doing. But if I replace it with a different behavior, if I ask something else of them, that redirects them really well and reinforces a new behavior.
>
> I'm just like those dogs.

When I asked what the experience itself was like, he replied: "Waves and blue and grey I remember. It was warm and pleasant and I liked the music."

This was actually huge for him, the beginning of a letting go, a quieting of the perfectionist producer mind he's been dominated by. This simple activity gave him the opportunity to rest in the experience rather than the analysis of it. In this preparation session, we talked about the need, the necessity, of making mistakes while being creative. Rather than squeezing the universe down into his expectations of what things "should" sound like, he wanted to be open to following its lead in discovering new ways of listening and playing. Because he was on tour during this session and was about to return to rehearsal, I encouraged him to take chances and allow himself to make mistakes.

For the third prep session, I asked him to listen to another piece of music, instructing him to let his imagination take off while feeling the song in his body. We were prepping him to relinquish control of the working mind, the default mode network, and place his attention elsewhere, where it was more in service of his heart's goals for presence and peace. This practice would help him tremendously during the psychedelic session.

He wanted to have the mental, emotional, and spiritual space to experience his life differently. These activities helped him be more fluid and easeful in his life and prepared him to navigate his psychedelic sessions with trust, surrender, openness, and curiosity.

I have detailed our preparation sessions so you can see that so much of the important work happens before a client even takes the medicine. This work alone changed the way this client played and recorded music. He was able to see and then release the perfectionism, and he started enjoying playing music again. Even before he engaged with the medicine, he told me his bandmates already saw significant changes, that he seemed to enjoy their gigs much more.

Fast-forward. How did this turn out for him? Well, if you would ask him now, he would say with childish delight, "I am finally drumming to my own beat." And, yes, I groaned too.

DEALING WITH EXPECTATIONS

Intentions are not expectations, and vice versa. Expectations are like entitled demands we place on ourselves, others, a situation, or the world itself. Usually, unmet expectations lead to resentment, dissatisfaction, and disappointment. I have seen too many clients come to the work with expectations masked as intentions. "I want to experience an ego death" and "I want to be happy" are two I hear often. This indicates there are unrealistic hopes and expectations of what the session, medicine, and therapy can accomplish.

I caution clients about the perils of holding expectations of the medicine because that is setting themselves up to be discouraged and it parallels how many people set unreasonable expectations of themselves in a way that reinforces the limiting belief that they are not good enough or are a failure. This is a great time in the process for clients to check the patches around success and self-worth placed on them in their youth. So much of our worth seems dependent on how we perform, and we project it externally, including onto the medicine therapy process.

Unreasonable expectations don't allow for spontaneity in the session and don't allow the medicine, therapy process, and the client's own wisdom to do their work freely. Again, so many are hoping for magic, which can, does, and will happen, just not the way we might expect.

Some people during session express disappointment and dissatisfaction, believing they are not doing it right, not seeing what they wanted to see, or not getting out of it what they want. I actually love when this happens, therapeutically speaking, because it showcases the expectations and beliefs that may unconsciously dominate them in their regular waking life, and we can address them right as they arise. Which part is arising, which core limiting belief is being exposed, how can inner wisdom, acceptance, and loving awareness intervene?

During the prep session, we also spend time exploring the subtle and subconscious expectations about "the magic bullet" that may arise in session. I counter expectations by helping clients create good intentions, by teaching them the COST stance (described in the next section), and by introducing the concept of the inner healer.

COST STANCE

As I reiterate throughout this book, "the medicine does what the medicine will." Once a medicine is taken, we cannot know or predict the experiences, memories, images, feelings, visions, insights, distress, or darkness that may arise. Although setting intentions is important, the truth is, once we begin the journey we are at the mercy of how the medicine works with our psyche, mind, and personality and within our brain.

COST stands for curiosity, openness, surrender, and trust. Although I encourage taking this stance for all sessions, it is especially important in the first medicine session, specifically for people who are new to expanded states of consciousness. Being curious and open as well as willing to surrender and trust sets the stage for exploring one's psyche and the cosmos with more ease because, if nothing else, we are learning to encounter the unknown with confidence, which ultimately helps us face the mysteries of our own life.

Curiosity

What is this? Why is this arising now? A black dragon is circling me . . . what does it mean? What's behind that door? Who is that standing on a cloud? Why is this memory showing up now? Curiosity is a mindset that counters fear. Fear says, "Hell no"; curiosity asks questions. It is relentless inquiry, like a child's mind, like having an inner Indiana Jones journey with us. Even when we are working with serious traumas, curiosity gives us a sense of wonderment at our own life and experiences as we go into medicine therapy. Curiosity challenges rigid black-and-white thinking, which keeps us bound to the very limiting beliefs we are hoping to let go of.

It's also okay to not know; to stay curious is to practice humility. Such a powerful practice for those of us who need to be the one who knows everything, to prove our worth by demonstrating invulnerability and false self-assuredness. In states of expanded consciousness, we can let go of those traits and enjoy the simple freedom of not knowing. It's actually quite refreshing and relieving to say "I don't know!" So freeing. Try it sometime, just say, "I'm not sure. I wonder. Maybe, who knows?"

First and foremost, be curious about and keep exploring what comes up in a psychedelic session. Be open to it all.

Openness

Willing, accepting, spontaneous, fluid, allowing, patient . . . this stance is about saying yes to what is, not shutting down. This willingness creates healthy ego strength, which suggests "I can do this. I can tolerate this." Being willing and able to sit with whatever comes allows access to deeper and hidden parts of the psyche that we usually shut down because it creates discomfort and tension. The door to the hidden treasure is usually guarded by dragons. We must face the dragon to gain access to what we are seeking. Practicing being open to whatever arises in session cultivates a willingness to try new things outside of therapy, to say yes more often.

Surrender

When the medicine hits, we want to let it take us where it will, to give up our control. Those who fight the experience often spend time working on letting go, which in itself is a healing and therapeutic practice. So there is nothing wrong with struggling to surrender because it points to our propensity to hold tightly and for our need to feel safe. Those who can surrender, or practice surrender, tend to be able to do the therapeutic work that often comes after fighting the experience.

This is especially true when using strong medicines such as 5-MeO-DMT, where the initial onrush is so strong that it strips the ego of its hold. Those who quickly surrender to the experience often find the wonderment, awe, and bliss they are seeking. When we surrender, we stop fighting reality, even if it is the reality of expanded consciousness and psychedelic states.

SURRENDERING

Try this on.
> First, bring your attention into your body. Feel the body's sensations.
> Then take two slow, deep breaths.
> Imagine floating on a gentle flowing river with your eyes closed.
> Allow your body to be taken downstream, moving with the current.
> Like a floating leaf, you are moved down the river, around rocks, swirling into and out of eddies, back into the main current.
> Gently be led, nothing to do but drift down the river.
> Let go.

(You can practice with me by choosing "Surrender Meditation" on my website, found here: www.michaelsapiro.com/meditations.)

What was that like? Could you feel your body relaxing, drifting? Did you tense up and want to get off the river?

I often ask people to imagine this as a way to experience surrender. Letting the current take us where it will.

This practice can be medicine itself because we often try to control so much of our life to feel safe. In practicing surrender, we become less rigid, less tense as we let life live itself.

Trust

As I discuss later, trust is crucial for the journey. I advise clients to trust that whatever arises is for their greatest benefit. Trust the therapist and space holder. Trust the medicine. Trust that the process and protocol are right. Trust that they are safe to let go and fully surrender. Trusting anything other than one's self is *so* difficult for traumatized people. Working on trusting is healing in itself, and so scary. It's hard to let go of the steering wheel, especially while driving, hard to believe another has our back, hard to close our eyes, hard to put our body into another's care, hard to open our consciousness to the universe.

I can hear many of you going, "Oh hellll no." Well, what are you going to do, remain committed to the belief that no one or nothing is trustworthy? That you have to do this alone? That mind frame will keep you isolated and in perpetual, constricting distrust. Part of the COST stance helps us practice trusting again. Even just being open to the idea is encouraging a new way of being. Learning to trust ourselves as we prepare to enter the temple of our own soul might be the most important element of rebuilding trust we can practice. When we learn to hear and trust the voice of our soul speaking, we find our innate wisdom and our inner healer.

INNER HEALER, INNATE HEALING INTELLIGENCE, AND THE MEDICINE DOES WHAT THE MEDICINE WILL

Just as the body begins to repair itself the moment an injury or wound happens, so too does our consciousness and psyche do the same with psychological and spiritual wounds. We just don't think about healing psychological wounds this way, though. Depression, anxiety, and trauma first and foremost are clusters of symptoms that are felt in the body and that affect the quality of our thoughts and our life. These physiological and mental responses are the way the brain, body, and nervous system send signals (symptoms) to our waking consciousness to let us know that something is not in alignment. When we avoid, repress, deny, push away or down, self-medicate, or numb these unwanted symptoms, we actually miss the very cues and clues that something is amiss. These very uncomfortable and sometimes unbearable symptoms are actually pointing directly to untreated and untended psychospiritual wounds.

The body and our consciousness possess an innate healing intelligence that immediately starts working on diseases, injuries, traumas, and illnesses. Sometimes both body and mind need extra support in the form of medical and psychological treatments and interventions, which work in partnership with our innate healing intelligence to create the best conditions for healing. I often say that our own wisdom is medicine because it provides insights, clarity, and the needed discernment to help us heal core wounds and to transform. This innate wisdom, which arises when the mind has slowed and becomes quiet, is also known as our inner healer. During psychedelic psychotherapy, when the ego cannot hold on to itself and rapidly dissolves and re-forms, we start to hear the wise voice of our soul. We hear the messages and truths that were drowned out by the voices of our dread, self-pity, worries and woes, fears, rage and resentment, and self-hatred and criticism. The inner healer has been waiting patiently for your attention, for the space to arise, and for you to hear it. Once it's heard, we can form a long-lasting loving relationship with the wisest and most compassionate part of ourselves.

Both the inner healer and our innate healing intelligence have been working on our behalf the whole time. It might just take someone or a psychedelic experience to bring them to our attention. That is what clients and I begin to do during the prep sessions. I encourage clients to pay attention to the signs and signals of healing working below conscious awareness. I want them to start to form a relationship with both their inner healer and their own innate healing potential so that after the sessions they can more easily integrate these wise parts into the whole. Doing this during psychedelic psychotherapy increases the likelihood the client can access and integrate their inner healer in the future. Imagine feeling psychological or emotional distress and then something inside you automatically points out the causes and suggests ways to work through it skillfully?! "You get to a point in your practice where the heart tells itself what to do," said Buddhist teacher Ajahn Chah, and this is what he meant.

And then there is the saying "The medicine does what the medicine will," which is a part of surrendering ourselves to the potency and transformational potential of the medicine. We can set our intentions and have a clear sense of what we want to work on, but the medicine and our inner healer (innate wisdom) will do what they want with us! So many clients feel surprised by what they've shared in session. Many share secrets they've been guarding. Repressed memories arise to be witnessed and worked on. So much of the material in psychedelic psychotherapy comes up unexpectedly as we are shown what needs to be addressed and processed. Don't let this scare you, though; this is actually what you need! Some of the most therapeutic moments come when we unexpectedly remember experiences, situations, and circumstances that have shaped our consciousness, personality, behaviors, and even the direction of our life.

Because we cannot really plan for what arises, we can rely on the COST stance to prepare to greet, welcome, and heal these buried or hidden memories and experiences. Unless I am asked specifically to bring up traumas or to redirect clients to their intentions, what arises is out of our control. And we want to honor this and the process of the mystery unfolding. We don't always get what we want, but we generally do receive what we need.

PREPARING TO ENTER THE TEMPLE

Although we may not consider psychedelic psychotherapy to be ceremonial in a traditional sense, we are doing deeply sacred work and thus I ask all my clients and retreatants to come to the work with a sense of reverence and respect, and I agree to do the same. We must treat each session, journey, or retreat as an important event, one that could very well save or transform their life. And we never know when we might meet God, so it's best to prepare just in case! Because this is sacred work, I invite people to prepare their body and mind as if they are entering a temple. This means reducing or eliminating the use of alcohol, marijuana, and other recreational drugs before sessions, which is important neurologically as well as personally because alcohol and other recreational drugs can interfere with the mechanisms of neurotransmitters and decrease the psychedelic medicine's efficacy and impact. Also, reducing or eliminating any habits that might actually be poor coping strategies and defenses increases the likelihood that deeper depressed or numbed feelings, images, and memories may finally rise to the surface of consciousness, where they can be welcomed and worked with therapeutically. I also encourage healthy eating habits and gentle exercise the week leading up to the sessions. The body and the health of the body must be included in our work.

I ask clients to groom themselves on the day of the session to prepare their body and mind to engage in healing work. How many of us rush through our grooming process, missing the chance to be with ourselves in a way that is nurturing and intimate? Most of us are so disconnected from ourselves we often have no idea what our body looks or feels like. When we prepare for a therapeutic psychedelic session, we want to slow down and open our awareness to our senses, breath, and being. This mindfulness is a good primer for what we will be doing during the session. I encourage clients to be mindful when showering and cleaning themselves. Smell the soap, feel the lather, sense the water droplets. Care about your body. Prepare yourself as if you're meeting your bride or groom on your wedding day or a goddess in a forested grove or your own inner radiant soul. Show up clean and ready to greet your own sacred heart.

Finally, I encourage clients to journal the morning of the session and to meditate. I often send clients my own recorded meditations or those of Tara Brach or Richard Miller, to name a few teachers I like.

STEPPING INSIDE THE TEMPLE

During this session, I have to prepare clients for the possibility of having an "ego death," which is when the ego dissolves so quickly that people can become disoriented and even terrified. Those who identify so strongly with their fictional ego can become frightened that they are the one dissolving or dying. But have no fear, it's not *you* dying! It's just the persona you thought you were!

This dissolving and the fear associated with it are totally normal, to be expected, and a sign that things are happening. I actually encourage my clients to allow themselves to die in this process (metaphorically speaking, of course!): "Let yourself die, then! Let go! See what awaits you." I want them to taste the freedom of being—pure being—because we are awareness itself. Life lives through and around us every moment, and we are not bound to our conditions.

When a new client shows up with no previous experience of altered or nonordinary states of consciousness, it can be difficult to give them an idea of the wide variety of experiences they may have during a session. It is like trying to explain what Thai food tastes like by handing someone a menu!

So how can we prepare ourselves for a potential experience of death and rebirth or for a mystical experience? And how can we make the preparation itself therapeutic?

The answer to both is trust, and in building trust, trust in our capability to handle whatever arises. Trust in our self is one of the most important factors of growth we can experience, so preparing for a therapeutic psychedelic session is preparing for life.

Then there is trust in the medicine, the process, the healer, and the mystery of life.

I often lead my clients in a very specific trust-building and surrender-oriented meditation to prepare for entering the psychedelic experience. (If you'd like to be guided through this, please visit my website and choose "Falling and Floating" at www.michaelsapiro.com/meditations.)

When we have established trust, we can more easily enter into a novel situation with confidence and surrender to what arises, even if the going is tough and even when we are scared or nervous when we start.

IT'S OKAY NOT TO BE READY

Please know, you don't have to do this right now, or at all, and until you actually take the medicine, you can back out or wait. This process is not for everyone, and you have to learn to listen to and trust yourself. If you are hearing or feeling a "no" within you or your body, listen to that voice or feeling.

It's certainly healthy to have some trepidation, fear, nervousness, and apprehension before engaging in psychedelic therapies, but if there is a strong message that it is not the right time or that this is the wrong process for you, please respect yourself. You don't have to give a reason or justify your feelings to anyone. "No" is a complete sentence. Too many of us have not been respected when stating our needs, so let this be a chance to advocate for yourself. You deserve that!

I believe preparation can be just as healing as the actual psychedelic session. I find that when done well, deep prep sessions deliver relief just by bringing hidden things to light. The prep sessions may leave us feeling raw and vulnerable, but we want to get to the heart of the hurt as quickly as possible, to bring into the light what has been avoided, repressed, numbed, and hated on. I find it best to bring the core wounds to the mind's surface as quickly as possible before we engage in the psychedelic experience, because that's what the medicine is most likely to do anyway. I want to bring those false messages and lies we've been told about ourselves that we believe in and reinforce through our unskillful and unhealthy behaviors into the light of our loving awareness, where they begin to lessen their hold over us.

The informed consent process, discussing and preparing for the psychedelic experience, letting go of expectations, discovering one's inner healer and innate wisdom, learning about the COST stance, and having permission to change one's mind are also important pieces that help clients have a sense of agency and autonomy over the process. This alone is healing and promotes empowerment and self-confidence.

CHAPTER 6

TRUTH MEDICINE
IT'S GO TIME!

I believe discovering, speaking, and living our truths, along with unconditional self-love, are the true medicines for our wounded hearts and traumatized bodies. Psychedelic psychotherapy helps us access both. This chapter walks through the actual process of psychedelic psychotherapy, but, first, some caveats: Each session is different, so though the details I offer are good basic handrails, know that, like any kind of therapy, the actual process and results depend on each individual person. Also, this is a rapidly evolving field, and other therapists may use a different protocol. The process I share here follows a basic structure, and this will give you a framework for what to expect.

The truth can arise at any time during the whole therapeutic process—during prep sessions, psychedelic sessions, and integration. The hope is that discovering, speaking, and living by our truths becomes a healthy normal habituated response, not just something that happens during psychedelic psychotherapy. However, to do this consistently, we need to turn truth-speaking into a practice, and that is explicitly what we are doing in psychedelic psychotherapy.

The realizing and releasing of truth evoke so many responses during a session: anger, grief, sadness, joy, elation, excitement, and hope, to name a few. What I almost always witness is relief—relief to finally have said the thing that needed saying—and then empowerment arises after. That is the feeling of strength filling the body from a clear, grounded heart that knows itself. The truth rings like a bell and resounds throughout the body. Besides unconditional love, which is the best medicine of all, speaking one's truth is a powerful healing balm and strengthening elixir.

The medicine itself, whether it is ketamine, psilocybin, or MDMA, is a core component of the experience because each works on different neural pathways and with different neurochemistry to create a vast array of subjective, phenomenological experiences.

Any substance that dramatically changes ordinary states of mind into altered states of consciousness unlocks vast portions of the unexplored psyche, and this takes courage to undergo. I have immense respect for every client who wants to heal and grow enough to participate in psychedelic psychotherapy with ketamine, psilocybin, or MDMA. (Not all medicines are appropriate for psychotherapy but may be very good for other types of nondirective therapies and ceremonial uses.)

Let's move on to the actual process.

In my work, there are five phases to a session: intro and grounding, onset, therapeutic exploration, the comedown, and the wrap-up.

A NOTE ON NOTES

I take journey notes on a laptop so the clients have their experiences and insights recorded and can read over them after the session. I record what they say and my responses or questions, which I put in parentheses to differentiate who's speaking. If a client talks a lot during a session, I may not be able to write down everything they say. In that case, I may paraphrase or allude to a longer story they shared.

I began this practice of note-taking when clients reported they struggled to remember what they shared with me and that it was difficult to follow through on their journal and integration assignments. The detailed journey notes allow them to journal and reflect more deeply on the therapy session and its impact. Depending on how high the dose, some clients even express surprise and wonder at what they said. Having notes, the client can also reflect on any signs, symbols, images, and metaphors that arose during the session and what, if any, meaning those images may have for their healing or growth.

DAY OF . . .

Intro and Grounding

Because of the extremely variable outcomes someone can have during a psychedelic session, a good therapist helps the client prepare for a variety of experiences the day of. I usually begin with a reminder about the COST stance—curiosity, openness, surrender, and trust—then we have a short discussion about their overall healing goals and the intentions for this particular session. I then lead them in a short grounding mindfulness practice.

Facing the unknown is a powerful practice. I use the time before the onset of the medicine to work with any of their fears and anxiety and to help strengthen their resolve to face the unknown with courage and trust. In a therapy session, we purposefully move toward what scares us the most, which is usually what we've been running from the whole time. This is good medicine in itself, and we should be conscious and aware how we face these minutes before departure. I often find data pertinent and relevant to a client's healing in the moments before the medicine starts working.

Remember, part of the work of both therapist and client is to pay attention—to attend to the signs and signals of the inner experience coming into awareness.

Onset

Strange new feelings and sensations can arise: floating, sinking, disappearing, dissolving, growing, shrinking, expanding, and contracting.

Old predictable ones can arise too: nausea, anxiety, the shakes, pain, exhaustion, or exhilaration.

The strength of the onset is medicine- and dose-dependent. Each medicine evokes different experiences, and even the same medicine on a different day can have entirely different effects.

This coming on can trigger a variety of emotional responses we want to attend to and take note of; it is all important information. How the client handles novel experiences during a session under the influence of a medicine can be indicative of how they may handle themselves during new situations in their normal life. As a therapist, I observe and attend to everything.

Therapeutic Exploration Phase

In the exploratory phase, we examine everything that comes up and arises in their consciousness. Images, sounds, shapes, textures, sensations, stories, memories, emotions. Doors, fields, stars, space, pyramids, forests, tunnels, catacombs, coffins, insects, trees, father, mother, sister, aunt, basements, creatures known and new. Not everything has meaning, but we must explore and discover what does.

The client is the explorer of the cosmos and their own psyche. The therapist is a guide, a psychological surgeon, a trusted friend, a confidant, and an attendant in this process. Good exploratory questions are essential here. These don't always have to be therapeutic, but they do help the client deepen their relationship with what is surfacing in the present moment:

> Where does that door lead?
> Where is the train going?
> What is it like being a marshmallow?

What does that memory mean to you?
Why is that coming up now for you?
Where do you feel that in your body?

Sometimes the meaning is obvious. Personal memories surface and demand to be acknowledged. One man in his thirties came for our ketamine protocol to deal with how his PTSD symptoms were affecting his relationship. He was scared in almost every situation, always worried the worst was going to happen. During the first session, he was hesitant to talk about his parents, simply saying they were good to him and he didn't want to speak badly of them. To me, this is always a sure sign the truth is being partially spoken but mostly hidden. My job is to encourage a deeper exploration of feelings about our younger years, the time when we were most obviously programmed by our caregivers. He said his mom worried all the time and he didn't want to worry his mom more by stating his needs or by doing things his way.

During his second session, he started to recall what it was like living with his father, who was a Marine. When he was around ten years old, his father would make him spar and wrestle, tactical drills essentially, to protect himself, to avoid being "taken by surprise" or, worse, "hostage." This was not martial arts training but rather punishing preparation in case the worst happened. Dad said it was bound to. So be prepared.

Think about that. Being ten and being physically forced by your father to prepare yourself to fend off people trying to abduct you. How would that affect your sense of self, safety, and trust in others?

He started to see how, from a very young age, he was being programmed by his father, and his mother who allowed this training to happen, to see the world as dangerous, to always be prepared for the scariest and worst kinds of danger. (Even later when he cognitively realized he would most likely not ever be in such scary circumstances, his body and brain continued to reinforce those original messages, keeping him on constant alert.) After three sessions, he was able to hold love for his parents but also speak to his anger and his utter dismay at being raised that way. He began to regulate his own nervous system and change the initial programming so that he could see the world as it is, not as his father had trained him to see it.

Sometimes in session feelings and images seem random but turn out to be significant. A woman in her thirties suffered over half her life with agoraphobia and panic attacks. She could barely be around people for fear of being embarrassed about something she might do "that was dumb or stupid." This fear kept her from socializing and from engaging in activities outside her home, and she struggled just to leave her house. During one ketamine session, she said she was being smothered by a marshmallow. She struggled to breathe and felt panic coming on. I guessed that this was what it must have felt like to live with agoraphobia and that intense fear of being scrutinized and judged. She immediately understood this to be true for herself. I asked if she could find the edges and look beyond the marshmallow. She said there was vast space, with stars. I asked how it felt. She said freeing and calming. I asked where the marshmallow was, and she said it had shrunk down to a small spot in her awareness. I encouraged her to continue changing the scope of her awareness, from the suffocating feeling to the greater sense of spaciousness.

Days later she reported that while standing at her refrigerator she felt the usual feeling of panic arising but then she opened her awareness to the whole kitchen around her. She immediately calmed herself and realized she was safe. After three ketamine therapy sessions, she went to a concert, then to a friend's party, and signed up for a 5k race. These three activities are a huge success for someone who could barely leave her home without panicking. She continues to struggle with anxiety but now knows how to care for herself while moving toward what helps her thrive.

The psychedelic psychotherapy experience can be many things—exciting, frightening, confusing, frustrating, complex, simple, full, and empty. One role of the client is to be an explorer and to simply be curious, open, trusting and to surrender (remember the COST stance) during the process. One role of the therapist is to help the client make sense of the experience and the material that arises during the journey in relation to the client's transformational goals and intentions. However, the medicine does what the medicine will, so we must remain open to where the medicine and the client's wisdom and intuitive senses take us.

One client, a firefighter in his forties, thought he was coming in to process some very difficult and traumatic critical incidents during his service. Instead, during the ketamine sessions, he talked about his father and grandfather. His mind expected to talk about one thing, and his heart shared something of more importance. And it turned out, the way he had been dealing with his PTSD symptoms (the fear responses, especially) was heavily influenced by the way his family taught him to see men feeling fear.

Most of our time together was spent processing the inner torment that arose for him as he tried to meet his father's and grandfather's unreasonable and unrealistic expectations about achieving and producing and what it meant "to be a man." His poor self-esteem and his overly critical self-judgments were created in response to thinking he was not living up to others' expectations of him. He could not, and would not, love himself because he saw himself as a failure.

We spent the first session talking about this, and he was open to the idea of loving himself and not being at fault for not living up to others' unreasonable and unrealistic expectations. He began to see the programming, what patches he wore. In the second session, he learned to put his hand on his heart and breathe in deeply when he was feeling scared (which previously meant he was failing and was paired with shame). He began to tell himself he was allowed to be scared at times, that it was natural and healthy. In the third session, he began telling himself that he loved himself when he put his hand on his heart. He realized he wanted to spend more time with his kids and to stop trying to prove himself. He was learning what his own heart-centered values were and wanted to commit to them.

Somatic Awareness During a Session

During a session, clients experience so many sensations and feelings in various parts of the body. Many sensations are just the normal pings and pangs of life, normal sensations that usually occur outside of our consciousness. Others, though, are connected to and represent memories. These sensations then become dharma gates through which we explore unhealed events. The body contains immense wisdom and needs to be listened and attended to, especially when the dominating ego can no longer control or repress the body's messages. In sessions, we learn to recognize somatic messages that hold important information for our healing. This is a model for how we can better relate to the body when not on a psychedelic medicine.

Signs, Symbols, and Metaphors

As discussed in more detail in Chapter 8, the subconscious speaks in images, signs, symbols, and metaphors. These may be ancestral, connected to a cultural or family tradition. Or religious or spiritual iconography or images can surface. Although they are not always interpretable in the moment, it is important to take note of these kinds of images and pay close attention to them as they arise. Sometimes we talk about them in depth as they relate to a client's healing or growth, and other times I just take notes for the client to reflect on after the session.

Overall, this is a time for the client to go with the flow and for the therapist to judiciously but thoughtfully ask questions and help make sense of the material and experience in relation to the client's healing and growth goals.

THE GREAT DISSOLVE: LIFE BEYOND THE EGO'S EDGE

The experience of the ego dissolving can look and feel like many things and take many forms. And as these experiences subside in session, we begin to process who the client is beyond the confines of their limited ego and what they learned in that expanded state. Then we apply it to their healing.

Sometimes You Lose Your Identity Completely

Are you a bird's song, a raven's wing, a tortoise shell with the world on your back? Or maybe you are a spinning dervish circling around planets in the vacuous space of infinite timelessness.

Maybe fear rises at first, then you hear me suggest: Go with it, surrender, let go, there's nothing to hold on to.

You let go and dissolve.

Maybe you become everything at once or nothing at all, just stardust.

And maybe you experience a freedom from suffering never felt before, *because there is no one left who suffers.*

There is so much to be gained from letting go of who you thought you were or who you were told to be. You can see yourself much clearer and see the bigger picture.

Now we look at your life, the traumas and challenges you brought in with you. You see new pieces you may have missed. You see yourself as you actually were back then. Why have you carried so much shame for what happened to you? You were so innocent. Awful things happen in life. Many of us have been hurt very badly by others. These untended wounds, traumas, depressions, and anxieties fill so much of our life and seep deep into our body until we can't stand it anymore. And yet, we are so much more than those precipitating events and difficult symptoms.

We do not have to live like this; this is not our natural state. The process of psychedelic psychotherapy gives us the much-needed distance to see clearly. It gives us more space internally so we are not so constricted by shame and fear. It gives us room to breathe.

COMING DOWN

This phase is about coming back to one's senses, often literally. We start to come back down from orbit in the cosmos or reemerge from the depths of the psyche into our body and our ordinary state of consciousness, and the timing here depends on the dose administered and our metabolism. But we now have new pieces to add to the puzzle of ourselves. Coming down almost always includes bringing back the gifts that we discovered during the session: Lessons, insights, new understandings, a widened sense of and deeper connection to self, and a whole new set of emotions contribute to the unfolding change that is taking place right here. We become aware of how our worldview and self-perception are shifting. The body feels different too: Senses are open and more vibrant.

I leave a lot of space for coming down. This is a time for quiet inner reflection, with some questions to help make sense of the whole picture. This is also a time for the client to become reacquainted with or reoriented to the physical body, much like an explorer might return to a warm home after an adventure in the winter woods. Many of us don't truly live in our body, just in thought bubbles. Having somatic experiences during a session helps us become more embodied and can remind us that our body can become a safe refuge where the mind can rest. This is a very important lesson for those of us with trauma, because we often feel afraid living in our own body.

The coming down can be a coming home. This, in itself, is such good medicine.

WRAP-UP: YOU DON'T HAVE TO GO HOME, BUT...

Actually, you should go home and rest! After the comedown, we talk about next steps, the do's and don'ts of aftercare.

Do's
- Be gentle with yourself, rest, and avoid overstimulation. Drink water and eat healthy, nourishing food, and if possible, spend time in nature.
- Reflect on your intention and how it showed up in your journey; take notes and journal about your reflections.
- Create two behaviors from your reflections. Small changes will create big results over time. A few common examples are as follows:
  - I will observe and stop negative self-talk, then be supportive and encouraging instead.
  - I will offer grace for making mistakes.

Don'ts
- Drive for the rest of the day.
- Watch TV or listen to overstimulating music that evening.
- Overshare with interested family and friends. It's okay to say, "I'm not ready to share about my experience yet."
- Draw any conclusions or make any big decisions without time to reflect on different interpretations and understandings of the experience—wait at least a few days.
- Drink alcohol or use other recreational drugs.

Wrapping up is not unlike seeing an old friend off after a long, meaningful visit. I share gratitude with my client and acknowledge the trust, courage, and vulnerability they showed during the session. If we have more sessions, I leave them with some reflective homework and daily spiritual practices to help keep the healing and growth going. If that is the final psychedelic therapy session, I prepare them for their integration sessions.

RETREATS

Here, I walk you through my typical retreat process, but know that every facilitator and organization has their own methods, and that these happen in locations where the medicines are legal to use. These are a few questions you should keep in mind to ask your facilitator before you embark on a psychedelic retreat:

- What lineage and training do the facilitators have and hold? How long have they been steeped in those traditions? What are their guiding philosophies and framework and orientation toward the medicine and this work?
- What does their tradition or training teach them about navigating difficult experiences? What is their policy on and practice with touch? How do the facilitators handle clients' distress? How do they ensure client safety during journeys?
- What does the integration process and post-retreat support look like?
- Have you, the potential client, vetted them? Is their program safe and well supported? Do you know others who have gone on this retreat before? How close is a medical facility if needed? It is ultimately your job to know as best you can what you are getting yourself into. Take the vetting task seriously!

The retreat process I've created is quite a bit different from my individual therapy sessions because I do not work one-on-one with the participants while they are on the medicine but rather help them open to the process before and integrate their experiences after taking the medicine. My team and I set the container for growth and healing in an extended workshop and meditation retreat format. As described earlier, before the retreat begins all retreatants are screened and then engage in prep work with a coach and on their own. These retreats generally run between four to six days.

The first night of a retreat is for bonding and establishing trust, setting intentions, and engaging in transformational exercises and meditation practices.

The next morning retreatants fast and groom themselves. We start our day with meditation, breathwork, and yoga. We have a fire ceremony in which participants offer what they want transformed and prayers and reflections of well-being for the group to the fire, and I read sacred poems. We offer our gratitude for the medicine, where it comes from and how it came to us, and ask that the medicine provide what is needed for participants' highest good and transformation. If we are using psilocybin, they take the dose then; if we are using 5-MeO-DMT, we guide the participants to their ceremony rooms.

For the psilocybin journey, everyone has their place set up in the shared space: mat, blanket, pillow, throw-up bucket (just in case), eye mask, electrolyte drink, and tissues. They may have pictures of loved ones or sacred items near them. Then they journey for three to six hours depending on the dose. The staff sits in the room with them on shifts, helping participants go to the bathroom, purge, cry, and work through difficult moments. In this role, we are caregivers, always monitoring and sending love into the room. Sometimes, our role changes to therapeutic support, helping retreatants process what arises in the moment or quietly encouraging participants to do their breathwork and go through the experience.

One by one, the participants come out of their journey and we encourage them to find a spot in nature close by the center to journal and reflect on their experiences. They are always in the staff's view. Later that night, we sit around a fire and share. This is when I lead a therapeutic group session, probing each for their insights and questions, using Socratic questioning to lead them to better understand their experiences and how their journey affected them. Then we usually have a healing soundbath to help soothe their nervous system and nonverbally integrate their experiences into their body.

The next morning, we begin again with fasting, grooming, meditation, yoga, and breathwork. If the medicine is 5-MeO-DMT, I lead trust activities to prime the group to surrender to this medicine, which can be quite intense. Participants are readied to surrender to the stripping away of their ego while being led by the medicine into mysterious and unknown places within their own psyche.

I do not engage in psychotherapy while they are on 5-MeO-DMT, but I do practice therapeutic questioning between "hits," and more specifically right after the last dose fades. Participants are very open and vulnerable during this phase and are more willing to talk about traumas and wounds. If they were lucky or courageous enough to move through the initial fear response and to surrender completely during the experience, they may have been gifted the experience of pure love. Many recount meeting God or the Divine during this time. After this experience, they remain in awe and wonder. Although this is not the "goal" of this type of session, it certainly is an incredible gift that can arise precisely because one was willing to completely let go and surrender.

That night, we engage in art therapy to nonverbally process and integrate their 5-MeO-DMT experiences; after dinner, I lead them through a therapeutic process where we verbally process their experiences. This is a very vulnerable and valuable time for the group to share what came up for them.

The final morning of the retreat is all about integration and what comes next, which I explain is the most important phase of this work. The integration phase begins that very morning talking about self-care and the psychological and spiritual practices they will have to engage in to sustain these new changes. After they return home, they engage in integrative coaching and are encouraged to enter into therapy.

A PROFOUND TRANSFORMATION

Individual sessions and retreats are so profoundly transformational for all involved. I have never seen a more powerful treatment, one in which it takes just a few sessions for people to find their truth, their voice, self-love and compassion, and their original innocent essence; greet their body; develop self-awareness; tend to their grief; and possibly release shame. Imagine experiencing just a few of these, how good it would feel. Now imagine being on a trajectory where you can discover most of these and sustain those feelings moving forward in your life. That's what psychedelic psychotherapy is.

CHAPTER 7

WHEN THE JOURNEY GETS TOUGH
NAVIGATING CHALLENGING EXPERIENCES

It is inevitable that difficult and challenging experiences will arise for both the client and the therapist during a session. If you decide to engage in psychedelic psychotherapy, you are allowed to struggle. There is no shame in what arises or comes out during a session. It is equally important for therapists to be skilled in dealing with their own internal responses while continuing to help clients navigate these difficult experiences with care, compassion, and tenderness. This work is about welcoming and accepting almost everything that happens in session (with exceptions of aggression, violence, or inappropriate sexual expression), not about avoiding difficult experiences.

At any given moment, the therapist must be aware of what is going on and how they will help navigate difficult experiences. I am constantly aware of what my client is going through as well as what I am experiencing in those moments, and if safety is not an issue or there is no imminent danger, how I can use whatever is arising for their benefit. Challenging experiences, though uncomfortable and sometimes distressing, can be so useful for pointing out underlying unresolved issues.

This chapter looks at three specific intersecting, interdependent processes:

1. What happens within the client
2. What happens within the therapist
3. What happens between the two

The difficulties that arise within and for the client are primary. The difficulties that arise within and for the therapist are secondary, but still important. The therapist should discern whether their difficulties are of an interpersonal nature and can be used therapeutically for the client's benefit or whether they need to be put aside to be worked on later by themselves. This is true of all therapeutic modalities but especially so during psychedelic therapies, when a client is in an altered state of consciousness and vulnerable.

Because psychotherapy happens on an intersubjective field, where the interpersonal component is such an important piece of the therapy and contributes to the meaning of the experience, it is essential that we also consider the difficulties that can arise *between* client and therapist.

The way therapists handle and help the client handle difficulties as they arise depends on what type of experience or challenge occurs. In my work, I use another four-domain matrix to assess where difficult experiences are arising: *physiological and somatic*; *psychological*; *spiritual*; and *interpersonal*. These domains are similar to the four domains I use during preparation.

Clients can experience difficulties in any or all of these domains at once, so it's helpful to have a way to quickly assess what is going on so I can be as supportive as possible. I'm sharing this explicitly so you know you are in good hands during experiences that might be uncomfortable, difficult, or challenging. As best we can, we want to be prepared for anything that can happen. Oftentimes, navigating distress in one domain leads to resolving issues in other domains. During the experience, the client must feel safe knowing they can trust their therapist to help take care of them and guide them through whatever difficult challenge comes up, if any. Then they can relax and surrender more fully, which is key to the success of the therapy.

Let's use throwing up as an example, which seems at first to be in the physiological domain for the client. But if we take a closer look, we can see how complex dealing with vomiting can be.

A lot of the time the purging is just bile, especially if the client fasted before the session and there are no contents in the stomach. Vomiting can occur because of dizziness or motion sickness (as with ketamine) or because the medicine upsets the stomach and encourages purging (as with ayahuasca and psilocybin). Generally, we handle this physiological response by having a trash can, towels, and maybe a warm washcloth nearby and offering some water.

If someone throws up, after I help clean them up, I look at the emotional, spiritual, or psychological contents of what was being purged. Was this simply a physiological reaction to the medicine, or did this occur in the context of bringing up traumas that live in the client's knotted belly? How could we use what was happening to lead us toward their therapeutic goals? I'm always assessing which domain we're working in, and they often overlap.

(On a very vulnerable sidenote: As a clinical psychologist, I was not trained in how to deal with this, so I had to learn as I was going. I had to learn how to tend to and clean the client, how to work with myself and my own "ewww, gross" response, and then how to become a tender mother or caring father. That became my role in those moments. Now I have no reaction other than to care for the client and maintain a therapeutic awareness.)

In this example, I would simultaneously need to handle my internal reactions, clean up and care for the client, help them feel healthy and safe, and then shift toward the mental or emotional content to work toward their healing.

In the spiritual domain, for example, the client may enter a psychic or cosmic realm they are not ready for. If the ego dies or dissolves, they may become frightened or hysterical at the sudden loss of "self." Some people scream loudly, and for long periods. In that instance, I might place a gentle hand on the client's shoulder, allow some space for the scream to be expressed, then coo or soothe the client. Then we can explore the experience together after it passes, which it always does. Distressing experiences can become the catalyst for understanding how their unresolved wounds and traumas continue to arise and play out in their life, because whatever we live with tends to come out during psychedelic sessions. But we work with this together.

I am not sharing these examples to frighten or dissuade you but rather to prepare you for distressing experiences you might have while engaged in psychedelic psychotherapy. Strange enough, they're almost always for your benefit, these challenging moments. You can learn a lot about yourself by navigating challenging experiences. Not only will you be cared for and tended to by your therapist, but you may also learn how to "welcome the unwelcome," as Pema Chödrön so wisely teaches, which is great training for encountering difficult circumstances in your normal waking life.

Patience, care, compassion, and skillful responses are needed on the part of the therapist. The client just needs to be curious, open, trusting and to surrender to the experience. That's so much easier said than done, for all of us involved! But this is what it takes to lead and be led through difficult experiences. Now let's take a more in-depth look into the four domains.

DOMAIN 1: PHYSIOLOGICAL AND SOMATIC

I make a distinction between the terms *physiological* and *somatic*. For me, *physiological* is anything to do with the impacts of the medicine on the physical body. Some examples of difficult experiences in the physiological realm are nausea, vomiting, shaking, elevated heart rate and blood pressure, sweats, fatigue, sleepiness, overstimulation, needing to urinate, overt sexual arousal, and psychomotor agitation.

Somatic refers to how the body responds to and expresses trauma, depression, anxiety, panic, and so forth. How does the body respond to psychological, spiritual, or emotional content? Where is it seen or felt in the body?

When I am observing a difficult physiological event, I differentiate between experiences related to the medicine and somatic expressions of something deeper. I work with these differently.

Some clients may have high blood pressure and so are concerned when taking ketamine; if this is the case, we have them on the blood pressure cuff and I watch the monitor. If I notice their BP is spiking, I may have the nurse add a medication that helps lower their blood pressure. This is one aspect of the physiology that I keep my eyes on. Psychologically, it may present as anxiety or emotional agitation. We must monitor our clients' bodies carefully because the somatic signs and the physiological symptoms may tell us something psychological or spiritual is arising or that there is an adverse medical reaction at that moment.

Although most therapists are not medically trained, everyone working as a psychedelic-assisted therapist or psychotherapist should have basic knowledge of how each medicine can cause physiological distress and basic safety and first aid skills. If you are considering engaging in psychedelic psychotherapy, be sure to ask about the therapist's safety plans and their training in handling any medical concerns that may arise in session.

Nykol Bailey Rice owns the ketamine clinic where I work. She is a highly skilled certified registered nurse anesthetist (CRNA) and psychiatric-mental health nurse practitioner (PMHNP) who is also trained in psychedelic science and therapy. This is an amazing and highly ethical combination of skills for someone who operates this type of clinic. The clinic is also staffed by other nurses, who are available to handle most medical and emotional issues that arise during sessions. At the retreats I lead for the special operations community, we always have on hand a nurse or a veteran medic to assist.

I have had to lead many clients to the bathroom, place extra blankets on them, apply a cool washcloth to their foreheads, and tend to their physiological distress or discomfort in so many more ways.

When I think of *somatic*, I expand the way I look at the physical body reacting to a psychedelic and wonder, "Is this a trauma or psychospiritual response?" Thinking somatically, I am curious about what is alive in the client's body in response to a memory, thought, or image. Is this freezing, arousal, agitation, contracting, or sinking related to how they experienced themselves during the original event or events? Somatic responses are clues. We can trace them back to their origin and right there apply love, compassion, soothing, or nurturing to the child, adolescent, or adult within who needs the most attention.

We are finally at a place in modern medicine and healing modalities, as a result of the pioneering research in the fields of psychoneuroimmunology and biomedicine, where we know without a doubt that the mind and body are not only interrelated and interdependent but also different aspects of the same organism. Of course, ancient wisdom and medical systems such as Ayurveda and Traditional Chinese Medicine, to name just two, already knew this. The mind–body interdependence becomes so clear in psychedelic psychotherapy when we witness physiological responses to internal stimuli such as thoughts, memories, images, and ideas. Our body not only keeps the score but also reenacts the same responses that occurred years, if not decades, before.

Do you find yourself confused by your body's response to stress or to joy? When was the last time you really listened to and investigated your body when in conflict? When have you checked in with your body as you made an important decision? Maybe these questions are as foreign as your body is to you. Psychedelic psychotherapy, as a somatically oriented therapy, can bring your attention to what is often ignored or denied, thus giving you immediate access to the wisdom of your body. This is no little thing. Most people live in thought bubbles rather than in the whole experience of themselves, which includes the body. Instead of ignoring the body's uncomfortable or distressing signs, which are actually signals that something is out of alignment, in PP we learn to pay attention and to tend.

This type of therapy is not the eat-greasy-pizza-and-take-an-antiflatulence-pill treatment that so many commercials try to sell you. This is a wake-up-and-mature process that helps you create a healthier relationship and bond with your body; sometimes during sessions, the body speaks loudly so you will hear. Although uncomfortable, it is an undeniable message that your body is alive and needs you to pay attention to it. These signals also point the way deeper inside to where memories are stored. Sometimes the most important gifts for your healing and growth come from awfully gross signals!

DOMAIN 2: PSYCHOLOGICAL

This domain is about the beliefs we hold about ourselves, others, and the world; our limiting beliefs, core wounds, traumas, and values we hold dear; and our relationships with our parents, caregivers, ancestors, community, and culture. The psychological domain includes our behaviors, thoughts, and personality style and traits. These features can arise at any given moment during a session.

Some examples of challenging psychological experiences may be the surfacing of deeply disturbing traumatic memories or fantasies, difficulty discerning reality from false memories, getting stuck in negative thought loops, and having to deal with difficult emotions such as fear, despair, and hopelessness.

On psychedelics, we can have extraordinarily difficult psychologically challenging experiences that are oriented around our beliefs about ourselves. "I hate myself. I'm a piece of shit." I have heard this sad sentiment so many times in my work. It's a core belief that discolors people's experiences, making ordinary daily activities bleak and dismal. Often, people pair their most basic and primal feelings with their trauma responses, making healing especially difficult.

I worked with someone whose son had committed suicide. He blamed himself for the suicide. Blaming ourselves for another's behaviors often arises from beliefs we hold about ourselves. Although this man intellectually understood that his son made this terrible choice as a result of his own suffering, he as a father *felt* responsible. "If I could have just supported him more instead of shaming him." My client's many "if only" thoughts kept him deep in his self-hatred. This made it difficult for him to grieve cleanly. From his shame and because he blamed himself for his son's death, he believed he deserved to feel bad the rest of his life. So, we spent most of our time identifying the underlying shame and self-hatred he carried before we addressed his grief, which had been untouched and unhealed for years. Once he saw that his self-hatred and shame were lifelong conditions that had been created in his youth, he could see how he had paired these responses with his grief. He could literally *see* this happening during his ketamine session. He saw his shame-self punishing himself. He began to choose redemption and grace and eventually felt compassion for himself not only for losing his son but also for the pain he experienced as a child. In his third session, he was able to grieve the loss of his son without punishing himself. Although at first his grief was huge and came out in torrents of keening wails, he was profoundly relieved and felt at peace for the first time in decades.

We often pair self-loathing, anger, or fear with our grieving, making it challenging to move through grief, which is a natural response to loss. So many of us suppress our grief, which often turns sour in our body as well as in our heart. PP helps us see all this clearly and address it.

Challenging psychological experiences must not only be navigated but also made sense of during or after a session. Everything in these sessions, including difficult experiences, becomes the very material that leads to our healing and release from suffering. Although we might not encounter challenges every session, it is imperative everyone is on the same page that these can occur at a moment's notice throughout the session.

The therapist must be extraordinarily skillful during these moments of vulnerability and treat the client and the stories or images shared as the most sacred material—because they are. When my clients truly feel safe enough to expose hidden secrets during a session, they experience great relief and lightness for having shared something never exposed or expressed before. From something challenging can come an end to the profound suffering from holding these secrets in.

Secrets

"I've never told this to anyone before" often precedes a client sharing the secret they've locked deep in their trauma vault or in the underground well of shame. I don't want to scare you away with the fear of revealing what you've hidden, but know that to fully heal means to look at all parts of yourself. In PP sessions, very little remains hidden from your newfound self-awareness. You have the opportunity to unearth and share your secrets so you can move on, forward, into the future without the shame that holds you back and down.

I can imagine you're feeling a bit nervous right now. Like, "Holy shit, I absolutely don't want to reveal *that thing!*"

Just know you are in charge of what you share. This therapy and these medicines are not truth serum or hypnosis. Your therapist won't make or force you to share anything. Your heart will do this for you, on your behalf, when it is ready. You are not sharing with the world or outing your most private information. This is between you and your therapist, who is (or should be) the safest container.

I can often sense when a secret is about to be shared. A client's body will tighten, they will steel their courage, which radiates into the room as strength. Sharing a secret takes so much courage and inner strength. Keeping one in "feels safer," but in the end, it is poison and eats away at us from the inside. And the pure relief when hidden things are shared is palpable! If I hadn't experienced this myself time and again, I wouldn't believe it either.

Remember Frank Warren and his *Postsecrets* art project mentioned earlier; there seems to be deep healing power in sharing one's secrets. Whereas the sharing in *Postsecrets* is done anonymously, it takes much more bravery to share a kept secret in the presence of another. Psychedelic psychotherapy can be the safe container in which someone looking for peace of mind and an open heart receives the inner invitation to reveal their scariest secrets.

In psychedelic psychotherapy, these secrets are witnessed and processed right as they arise and are shared. Because there is no moralism in this therapy, just pure loving awareness, compassion, and wisdom, the client often feels safe and free to share hidden information in hopes it provides deep relief and moves them closer to their intentions and goals.

The secrets I've heard are often mired in shame, embarrassment, self-loathing, confusion, fear, and judgment. Because we are already working with unconditional love, compassion, and clarity, revealing these well-kept secrets in session makes complete sense.

Sometimes the client is the perpetrator of harm, but more often than not, they were the victim. Both the causing and receiving of harm create deep shame that affects one's life in immeasurable and destructive ways. Other secrets are about longings, desires, fetishes, private habits and behaviors, and dreams for the future.

> ## YOUR SECRETS
>
> If you are feeling any emotions bubbling up while reading this section on secrets, please know you are not alone. If you could shadow me for just one day, you would see how common it is for us to keep secrets that fuel our shame. This is true for almost all of us. I hope knowing this might be the permission you need to begin or continue your healing journey more honestly, sharing what has been kept in the dark.

When I ask my clients what prompted them to share their secrets, they often respond in a similar fashion: "Well, I was already being so honest with myself that it was time to let that out," or, "I saw it clearly and thought, 'Let's just get it over with.' I've never felt so safe before." When the conditions are right, many clients feel safe and ready to share.

And to be clear, I do not solicit, provoke, or prime clients to share their secrets. This sacred material must be given freely, without pressure or manipulation. The impetus to share is so personal and the courage to do so is generated from the heart's deepest desire for healing and change. Any coercion takes away from this process of generating courage and empowerment, which can then be used in normal, waking life. What greater gift to give one's self than confidence and empowerment?

Many of us believe that some secrets should go to the grave with us—just out of pure "self-preservation." However, I've witnessed and have experienced how sharing secrets in this process is freeing and relieving, because secrets provide the context for a lot of our suffering and harmful behaviors. Just some food for thought!

Note that because licensed therapists are mandated reporters, we do have a legal obligation to report any of the conditions specified by law. This must be discussed during the informed consent process. And, yes, even while under the influence of a medicine and in an altered state of consciousness, clients are ultimately responsible for what they share. Skillful therapists can stop a client's sharing at any time to remind them of these limits of confidentiality and ask whether or not they want to disclose these types of secrets. Complex, isn't it?! For your peace of mind, in my experience, navigating this type of difficult experience is very rare.

DOMAIN 3: SPIRITUALITY

This domain is about meaning and purpose and our connection to ourselves, others, and the world. It covers our beliefs in God, universe, the divine, emptiness, the void, everything and nothing. Spirituality focuses on how values are based on these beliefs of our connection to what is around and within us. It includes how we relate to our bodies, whether as meat suits or as "divine vessels" that are as important as our consciousness.

Spirituality also has to do with spirits, ancestors, energy, and nature. Psychedelic medicines seem to open us to more than we sense we are. And there are times in sessions when a client senses things coming into their space, into their field of awareness. Whatever that is can be a connection to the cosmos itself and can help them feel connected to the greater universe and to their own lineage of ancestors. Are these created by the brain or do they come through the brain? To be honest, I don't really care. What is perceived while in an altered state is real to the perceiver. How we make sense of and use that material for our own good and well-being is of utmost importance to our healing and transformation.

Spirituality is within and beyond our personalized ego and our individual self. The spiritual realm is infinite and is often not brought into the field of medicine in the West. However, because of psychedelic therapy, we are starting to fuse spirituality with healing because it is a core component of our human experience. Our connection to the divine, God, mystery, Source, ancestors, Earth, energy, and emptiness and form informs how we are in the world, and the data suggests that those who feel more connected have better health outcomes.

But what happens when "the shit gets dark" and confusing?

Making room for the complexity, the contradictions, and the paradoxes that we are is part of the work during sessions, especially when there are challenging spiritual experiences involved. All of us are wildly vast. We all include more parts of humanity and the universe than we could imagine. When we start realizing and experiencing that reality, it can be extraordinarily overwhelming and potentially destabilizing.

In the Bhagavad Gita, holy scripture from Hinduism, Krishna, a major god, teaches Arjuna, a warrior, about the nature of the universe, which is also Krishna's inherent nature. Arjuna says, "I really want to know you. I want to know about the nature of the universe," and Krishna says, "Are you sure? It's going to blow your mind and scare you." So Arjuna is like, "No, no, I can do it." Krishna unleashes the cosmic forces and unravels the fabric of the universe for Arjuna, and Arjuna's mind is blown, and he says, "Shut it down! I'm good, I get it!" It's way too much for the human mind to comprehend.

In many mystical and religious stories about a person meeting or seeing the face of God, the person usually goes mad. At least at first. When clients come into contact with the infinite textured layers of themselves that arise from a vast formlessness, which is understood to be the Source of all things, there is often destabilization of and then dissolution of the self. Welcome to a potential spiritual experience in psychedelic psychotherapy!

Our mind (and brain) needs coherence and to be selective in its attention in order to make our existence "simple" and streamlined. If we are perpetually aware of the complexity of all internal and external stimuli and sensory input at the same time, we could not function. As mentioned, many psychedelic substances disrupt the brain's default mode network, which contributes to their also increasing the entropy of brain signals and thereby altering our "normal" sense and perception of reality. Don't worry, this can be good news! Practically, an increase in brain-signal entropy is thought to mean that our "normal" way of perceiving things strongly based on expectations and beliefs is disrupted, allowing for more possibilities to arise (think of this as a freedom of mind). In neuroscience, increased entropy is generally associated with a disruption in fixed patterns of signaling and enhancement of new connections between and within brain regions. Deep meditation and spiritual and mystical experiences have been reported to have similar impacts on the brain and perception. So we must be prepared to navigate this potentially unsettling experience in session.

When a client starts unraveling and their mind and sometimes their inner and outer voices are screaming, "Oh my God, I never wanted to see all these things!" we rely on our established plan of returning to a place of safety, security, calm, and love in which they are held. Because I know that unraveling during a session is possible, I make an agreement with the client *during our prep work* that, if things become too difficult, we return to a place of calm respite and ease. Richard Miller of iRest calls this refuge an "inner resource," which is a feeling of safety and security that is evoked by first imagining what brings us calm and ease, and then internalizing that peace as a natural part of us. I teach this practice to my clients at the beginning of our first session so they get used to calling on their inner resources during challenging moments. We also practice deep breathing and placing our hands on our heart.

If the client is unable to handle the dissolution of their ego, and their experience is no longer therapeutic, we return to what is present. This is where directing an individual's attention back to their breath, body, and present-moment awareness is so helpful.

My job is to recognize when a person may not be ready to see the face of God or whatever spiritual material is arising and to guide them back to the room and to help them ground themselves and stabilize. Once that happens, we can talk about what just happened, and their frightening or destabilizing experience can become a therapeutic one. It is good data to know they may not be ready to face the parts of themselves they've been hiding, repressing, or denying their whole life. To me, any spiritual experience in session always points to the client's inner world. Whether spirits or ancestors appear, they see the face of God, or they disassemble into disparate parts of the cosmos, it is all happening within and highlights what is ultimately not integrated in their life.

Do ancestors come into the client's field and speak of traumas long ignored or forgotten by countless generations?

Do spirits or otherworldly entities with unrecognizable features and fantastic faces arrive?

Neither of these examples need to be considered difficult or challenging, and in fact they can be welcomed with a sense of openness and curiosity with the right preparation work. How do we skillfully navigate when potentially unwelcomed beings or entities arrive in session and evoke great fear or terror? What happens when what arrives or arises threatens our deeply held religious beliefs or our existence itself? Whether fictional, fantasy, or real, what arrives and arises must be seen as sacred information of the psyche and cosmos emerging and should be navigated with care for the sake of our healing and growth.

One of the primary differences between psychedelic psychotherapy and other forms of psychedelic therapy or ceremony is that the therapist and client begin to make sense of and use what arises right in the moment to better understand the client's inner world and to move toward healing.

Depending on the client's reaction or response, I may encourage them to continue exploring what's arising or what they make of it. One situation stays in the direct, difficult spiritual experience, and the other pulls the client back to a meta-level view of the experience. If their reaction is one of dysregulation that cannot be tolerated, we engage in grounding and returning to center.

When the client lets me know they feel stuck within the experience, I offer encouragement to engage with it if possible. Following are some prompts I may use when a client is faced with an unwelcomed presence:

> Maybe say hello?
> Can you communicate with it?
> Can you ask what they want or need?
> What messages do they bring?
> What do they look like?

A specific example:

> Can you sit next to your grandmother at the fire and see what that feels like for you? Can you ask her questions?

Here are a few prompts on the meta-level:

> Does this remind you of anything specific in your life?
> Why do you think this is arising for you right now?
> What does this make you want to do right now?
> How might you face this directly?
> How might you set firmer boundaries with it right now?

All their responses are useful for understanding not only the content deep within them but also how they deal with challenges, difficulties, and situations that seem scary in their normal life. I always keep in mind a client's initial intentions and therapeutic goals because those direct the types of questions and support I offer during the challenging experience.

Because it is a safe and supported environment, the container of psychedelic psychotherapy is a powerful place for a person to face the mysteries deep within with courage, openness, and curiosity, which pays off down the road in real life.

DOMAIN 4: INTERPERSONAL

Have you ever just not liked someone? Silly question; I know you like everyone you meet. I'm kidding! Of course you don't like everyone. Imagine finding out in the middle of a psychedelic therapy session that you didn't like your therapist, or worse, you as the therapist don't like your client! It happens. Normal relationships are complex, but when one person's consciousness is altered by powerful psychedelic medicines, interactions can become even more challenging.

This is the interpersonal realm. Inside the client, inside the therapist, and between both. How are you and I doing in session? Do you trust me? Do I trust you? What happens when attraction arises, one way, the other way, both ways? What happens when you feel repelled because this person is so much like your dad and you think, "I don't even want to be in this room with them."

Do I represent your dad, brother, lover? Do you represent a sister, mother, lover to me?

Do my ethnicity and gender play a role in a client's feeling of safety and trust?

Do my implicit biases unconsciously inform how I operate and direct my interventions?

These dynamics are ongoing and must be reflected on constantly for a few reasons. One, interpersonal dynamics are part of the undercurrent of the therapeutic process, and other times they are active waves. Two, these very dynamics can be used as data on what is going on in the internal worlds of both therapist and client and, most importantly, can be used in the service of the client's healing and growth.

A therapist is obligated and ethically committed to helping the client whether they "like them" or not. Therapists must quickly discern whether the feelings can be useful and helpful to the client in the session or they are for the therapist to work through on their own afterward. It can sometimes be helpful to let the client know how their behaviors are landing because we might have just uncovered a pattern that plays out often in their life. Bringing kind, therapeutic attention to a relational pattern that may push others away can bring clarity to a client and potentially be very healing.

Clients get to be honest and truthful during a session in a way they might not allow themselves during normal life. They can give feedback and discover whether their feelings arise because of something the therapist is doing that does not work for them or they are projecting based on their past. Either way, this "not liking" business can actually be very therapeutic and healing.

The healing comes when a client has the courage to voice what is felt to a therapist who can hold the tension and space to process. Maybe trust was broken. Maybe the client doesn't feel heard or seen. Maybe the therapist has done nothing but reminds the client of a parent or an ex. Although difficult in the moment, sharing these feelings can be relieving and empowering for the client.

All the same interpersonal issues that come up in traditional talk therapy can arise in psychedelic psychotherapy: transference, countertransference, projections, and projective identification, and everyone's attachment styles are activated too. Humans meeting other humans being human. It just happens one of them is on psychedelics. Complex, isn't it?

Almost all the client's behaviors, thoughts, and words about a therapist are data that can be navigated and used to move toward a therapeutic goal. Even in the most difficult interpersonal experiences, I know all the client's behaviors are ultimately about them. I do my best not to take anything that is happening personally. And if I find myself not liking the client, for whatever reason, I know it is ultimately about me and then work to return my attention right back to the client. I trust that everything happening is arising in service to their healing and growth.

What happens when a client's negative personality traits and behavior style point directly toward the therapist? Or the client begins to sexualize or fantasize about the therapist? How does a therapist navigate when a client says, "I hate men, and you're a man. You're trying to manipulate me. Why are you gaslighting me?"

Sometimes the work in these situations is about having a corrective experience for the client, demonstrating that the therapist can "handle" them when others might have rejected or moved away from them. Other times, the therapist must set firm yet kind boundaries and return the focus to the client's experience.

The most important therapist response is maintaining a stance of compassion, equanimity, and nonjudgment, avoiding shaming the client in any way for their behaviors but using those very behaviors to point back toward their inner experience.

"BAD TRIPS"

I am an outspoken proponent of the idea that there are no bad trips. Now, before you go yelling at me with all your horrific psychedelic stories, let me explain myself. I know there can be very, very scary, difficult, challenging, and disturbing journeys and painful physiological responses while on psychedelics. I do believe, however, that many of these experiences can be useful for healing and growth when the experience is understood in the context of a person's life and is supported in a healing and safe environment.

"Bad trips" are really experiences that are not well prepared for or supported, or they happen in the wrong setting, when there is no one available to help someone who is scared, lost, or confused. The loss of ego can be frightening because by nature it is a destabilizing experience. (I am not talking about physiological or psychological reactions caused by contraindications to the drug itself. Again, not everyone should be using psychedelic medicines.)

So many clients think they want to experience an "ego death" and then when it happens they freak out! It's ironic in a way, because it's the ego freaking out that it is losing control of its hold on its host's consciousness. Pure, unconditioned consciousness is what many are seeking to experience but are not willing to allow their constructed sense of self to disintegrate to allow what's pure and original to be experienced.

When I asked a group of psychedelic therapy students to define what makes a "bad trip," they collectively came up with the following descriptions:

> It's uncomfortable, unsettling; resistance and fighting of the experience; creates a response with heightened emotions; triggering, creating pain and avoidance; anti-euphoric; reliving horrific traumas; facing difficult emotions based on one's life circumstances.

For me, this is all grist for the mill. It's what we can use during psychedelic psychotherapy to move toward our goals. In the moment these responses arise, we can direct our loving and compassionate attention to actually heal ourselves.

SAFETY

Safety of the client and the therapist is paramount and always needs to be considered first. However, people are unpredictable on drugs. And depending on the medicine, the higher the dose, the more likely a client may lose control of their behavior.

A trusted colleague and good friend called one night to debrief a situation in which one of her clients grabbed onto her, wrapping his arms and legs around her from behind. Though it lasted for less than a minute, this experience left her shaken and questioning herself as a guide and psychedelic therapist. The client had no memory of the event, which at first I did not believe, because it usually takes an extraordinarily high dose for someone to completely lose their conscious awareness during a psychedelic experience. It turned out, he'd asked for more during the session and she agreed to the increase in dosage. Increasing a client's dose during a session is not uncommon, but this time she allowed for an additional dose that left him in a blackout and her being threatened.

She was very lucky that he did not hurt her and left her only scared. We debriefed many topics, including her being alone with a larger male; her trusting the client to not become threatening because she knew him; her allowing a second dose that was much too high and unsafe for both of them. These considerations must be worked through before the session as best as possible, but unfortunately, the only way she could have known the answers was through this experience.

I have also learned many lessons the hard way, which is why I stress that my students seriously prepare themselves and train. Even a highly skilled and trained therapist cannot predict what will happen during a session. The more prepared we are to stay calm and have a whole toolbox of responses ready, the more likely everyone stays safe.

Although people may experiment on their own with a variety of doses, it is ultimately the therapist's responsibility to administer, and monitor, the safest dose for a therapeutic experience.

Safety-Health-Healing-Growth

Safety, health, healing, growth—this is the order when determining interventions during challenging experiences. My perspective is that most of the challenges that arise are navigable and can be used to further treatment goals.

Besides purely physiological difficulties, most of the challenging experiences arise from the client's psyche. This is what we want in psychedelic psychotherapy, not necessarily the challenge, per se, but the sacred and therapeutically important material that becomes exposed and that is brought into light. I want the client to know that it is okay, safe, and important that this material arises in session. Even the darkest secrets from the trauma vault need exposure to the light to be broken down, healed, loved on.

So many people avoid their emotional and psychospiritual pain so that when it is arises in session, and they finally have to face it, they can initially experience much distress. But when they face it bravely, they get through the distress and break through to healing. It takes so much courage to do this work, and I let them know this as the difficulty arises in the moment. Great benefits are possible when a client moves through this distress.

After my separation and divorce, I went through a personal hell that I'd created myself. For five years, I punished and hated myself, believing I was solely responsible for the dissolution of my marriage, even though my former wife never once blamed me. I believed I could punish myself into redemption, but after five years of that, it was more than clear I was only hurting myself. When I began to work on self-forgiveness, it took only about a month of *dedicated focus and practice* for this forgiveness to come to pass. (With the amazing guidance of my own depth psychotherapist. Thanks, John!)

Think about that.

I avoided something so good for me, something that would have brought me deep relief. Instead, I hated and punished myself for five years.

That's insane.

In this work, we face the dragon directly. For me, it was very difficult to forgive myself because I encountered so many harmful and limiting beliefs that prevented me from forgiving myself, beliefs that were not mine to begin with. I'd internalized others' beliefs that I had to punish myself, that I was not inherently worthy of forgiveness. I was so distressed seeing and feeling all this. But I persisted and kept doing the work.

Psychedelic psychotherapy helps us see not only what we are doing to ourselves and how we've held on to traumas and harmful beliefs but also how to let go and heal.

One of the retired police officers I worked with said she was afraid "to face the darkness." In one of our ketamine sessions, she arrived at the very place she had been avoiding for so long. She said, "I'm scared to go into this. Let's just avoid it. I'd rather go back to the water over rocks," which was a soothing image that she had been working with.

I said, "Yes, that's what you've been doing your whole career and into your retirement. And it doesn't seem to be working for you. How about we navigate your darkness together? Navigate what you're afraid of together?"

She had been living in and with fear for most of her life, through her career and now into retirement. Her avoidance and coping strategies were not working. Her intention was to learn to let go of her fear and live a life of ease and joy. Soothing strategies help in the moment but don't address the underlying causes of perpetuated fear. She was in ketamine-assisted psychotherapy to face the dragon. I reminded her of this in session: "How about we take the courage and strength you relied on as an officer into this session? Because doing this will transfer into your life outside of this session."

And she did.

While the ketamine worked on her nervous system and brain, the water and stones soothed her, and her own inner strength helped her face what she had avoided for so many years.

In psychedelic psychotherapy, the lasting effects of trauma, anxiety, depression, moral injury, untended grief, shame, and guilt can arise in any and all the domains discussed throughout this chapter. A psychedelic psychotherapist helps clients navigate the myriad of psychospiritual consequences caused by some of the worst experiences and traumas a human can go through or witness.

If you decide to engage in this type of therapy, your job is to show up and to be raw, vulnerable, authentic, and willing to face what you have avoided for so long, for the sake of your health and well-being and a thriving future that depends on this work. You are signing up to be fully present and alive in your own experience of yourself—maybe for the first time in your life. And this can be difficult and challenging but ultimately so rewarding.

SHOWING UP AS A THERAPIST—AND AS A COMPASSIONATE HUMAN

When I become uncomfortable in session with any of the difficult experiences mentioned earlier, I remember I am there as a nurturing person as well as a therapist. I am fluid between roles. I am also very direct as a therapist, especially when working with veterans and first responders (okay, with everyone I work with!). I speak directly to the harmful ways they are thinking or speaking about themselves and how their limiting and negative beliefs affect their lives. But if they are in serious distress, I adjust and offer soothing and tender care, which may include hand-holding or touching their shoulder (per our agreement on touch).

My ultimate commitment is to their well-being and I adjust as needed in session. As discussed earlier, a therapist's framework and orientation must be disclosed and discussed in the intake and prep phase of this work so that the client is aware and can consent to this style of healing interaction.

Bearing Witness Bears Fruit

Even though this book is about psychedelic psychotherapy, in which a therapist is actively involved during a client's psychedelic session, there are times when doing "nothing" and being a loving witness is the appropriate therapeutic response during a challenging experience.

One of the combat medics I worked with experienced a series of flashbacks in which he was in contact (engaged in combat) and his fellow Marines were being shot at and some killed. His primary job was to provide emergency medical care to any fallen brothers, and as the horrors of war go, many did not survive, which he held himself responsible for. In his psychedelic experience, he began rolling around on the floor screaming, "I'm so sorry. I'm so sorry I couldn't save you," processing his grief and survivor's guilt. He was rolling around, hitting the floor, crying and sobbing "I'm so sorry" for well over ten minutes.

This was a time for me to bear silent witness to his deep pain. He needed to express this in any way he could without interference. Because he was safe to roll around and there was nothing but love I could offer from a distance, I put my hand on my heart and felt deep compassion for him. Tears welled up in my eyes and I felt love and sadness for him for having witnessed his brothers die before him and in his arms. I felt compassion for all people around the world who suffer because of the seemingly unsolvable greed, hatred, and ignorance that fuel destructive wars that leave people terrified for the rest of their lives, including my own grandparents who survived the Holocaust.

He needed space and a witness to express his horror, grief, and love. As it subsided, I moved close to him and he reached out for me. I held him as he sobbed.

I can feel his presence, and these feelings, as I write this now.

Later, he was able to describe what was happening and the powerful lessons he learned:

> What I was reliving was an amalgamation of all the calls I was on. Both as QRF [quick response force], in direct action, and a sniper's ambushes over the course of two weeks.
>
> That experience brought back one I'd put out of my mind entirely. A VBIED [vehicle-borne improvised explosive device] outfitted with chlorine gas, which causes those exposed to essentially drown in their own fluids.
>
> They train us like we are all-powerful. Like we can handle any situation put in front of us. They build up our confidence in

control mechanisms, and we become the "gatekeepers." The reality is very different.

I carried the weight of not being good enough for so long. Yet, according to the paperwork, I was always one of the best. It tortured me that I literally couldn't work hard enough or be good enough. I couldn't find a way to be any better. That's what I was able to let go of in that experience. I learned that I AM good enough. That some things are simply in hands more powerful *than my own.*

Since that time, he has become an integration coach for other combat veterans who go on psychedelic retreats for PTSD, suicidality, substance abuse, and depression. He also acts as the medic on these retreats. His intention for his work is to "see the lights in their eyes come back."

Sometimes the best intervention is bearing witness and holding loving space for a person to express what needs to come out. It takes time, training, and experience for a therapist to build the skills needed to discern when to hold that space and remain quiet and when to intervene during challenging experiences.

Because these medicines open us to the great mystery of life, there is no way to predict or plan for specific challenges that may arise during a session. However, both clients and practitioners of psychedelic psychotherapy can prepare ourselves to be skillful explorers of the unknown.

CHAPTER 8

PSYCHE AND COSMOS
EVERYTHING, EVERYWHERE, ALL AT ONCE

She could smell smoke and asked if anything was burning in the room. On ketamine, her senses were sharper than mine, so I looked around to check. No, I assured her. Explore that and see where it takes you, I suggested.

She was in her thirties and working through severe childhood trauma, and she had the intention to connect to and heal some of the ancestral traumas in the long lineage of women who had suffered in her family. She wanted to be a different kind of mother to her daughters, and she knew she needed to heal from the damage of the violence done to her as a child to meet this goal.

Sometime in the second half of the session, she was transported to a forest and saw a fire with a shadow of a woman she couldn't identify.

I smell animal fur. It feels indigenous. My grandmother. I see her. She's rich with life. I can sense her, but not see her. I can sense her life. She's still here if I want her. She's heavy...

I can still smell animals, horses and mammoths. It's a dense fur.

This woman was so deep into her experience being with her grandmother in some primal setting that she could smell the wild. Therapeutically, we used this experience as a platform to further connect with her grandmother, whom she eventually met:

She has beautiful brown skin. Gorgeous red hair. She is calling me to sit with her.
I can see other women who fought and struggled for survival in my family.
They are so beautiful, so strong in their suffering.
They are telling me I can get through this.

Her hope was to heal what they carried as well as heal herself from the deep pains caused by the terrible abuses committed by her mother. All this to be a healthier, unconditionally loving, nurturing, and more present mother to her two young daughters.

Throughout the session, her psyche and the cosmos provided clues, scenes, and scents to help her connect viscerally and across space-time to what was living deep within her—all for transforming generational pain into her own strength and wisdom. She left that session feeling more connected to herself, her ancestors, and the greater world around her, which lessened her sense of being alone in her suffering.

Please understand that this is the beginning, nowhere near the end, of her healing. Seeing her grandmother or any ancient grandmother archetype gave her the strength she needed to face the dragon of her deepest wounds:

How could my own mother treat me that way? How could a mother throw a daughter down the stairs? How could she blame me for being sexually abused by her husband, calling me his mistress at twelve years old?

What's wrong with me? Am I really that bad? Did I deserve it?

These questions had prompted her to act out and harm herself through much of her adolescence and kept her spiraling into shame and pity for most of her life. These beliefs kept her from loving herself or even her daughters the way she longed to. Exploring her psyche and the ethereal world of the cosmos was a tool and a prompt on her healing journey.

(I imagine you are sitting with a lot of feelings for her, and maybe for yourself. Please take a moment to feel whatever is present, maybe breathe into your heart, and offer yourself, and her, compassion.)

Not every psychedelic experience or psychotherapeutic session leaves us feeling connected to ourselves, our ancestors, or the greater universe. However, the majority of people wisely using psychedelics and engaging in psychedelic therapies often report an increased sense of interdependence and connection beyond themselves while a deeper understanding of and relationship with their own psyche is established. This is essential for people who feel disconnected from themselves and their life, which I see as a major cause of depression. Exploring our psyche is essential for living authentically, from a place that is unique and original to ourselves, while feeling a sense of belonging to the greater whole.

When we slip into these deeper levels of consciousness, we are exposed to our personality, our core beliefs and wounds, our strengths and hopes, the interdependent nature of reality, and, yes, the tightly woven fabric of the cosmos itself. Images, symbols, metaphors, signs, and visions play a role in our healing and transformation. This is so valuable because we may be so disconnected from ourselves while making ends meet and weathering the stresses of living in such a fast-paced world, where bills are constantly due and chores need to be done. But being disconnected from ourselves is a major source of depression and anxiety. Connecting to, learning about, and truly supporting ourselves feels good, alleviates stress, and increases our well-being. We learn what we really like and want and become the force that moves us toward what is good for us. Isn't that what we are really looking for in the first place?

So many come to me not knowing who they are and feeling misaligned with the life they are living. Often during sessions, while exploring their own psyche and the experience of raw and unfiltered life, clients naturally begin to discover who they are and realign with their deepest and authentic values. Doing work on these levels also exposes the origins of so many harmful behaviors we get stuck in, making it easier to create sustained healthy changes in the process.

OUR SHADOW PARTS

When we first glimpse our depth during psychedelic psychotherapy, we often want to turn and run, because this is where our shadows, hidden parts, and wounds live. And this is exactly what we've been trying so hard to avoid in the first place! But it is also where our hidden talents, gifts, passions, brilliance, and genius live too, which we also miss when we avoid ourselves.

Remember when I mentioned the liberating power of truth earlier and how the *Postsecrets* project allowed people to express themselves and be seen? Going into our psyche and exploring the vaster cosmos is like that. It can be frightening at first to see ourselves and our interconnectedness in the raw. It takes courage to be this vulnerable. It also takes grace, compassion, and forgiveness to discover what's hidden. Psychedelic therapy gives us awareness, which allows us to heal what we discover—and more importantly, to see ourselves in our wholeness.

THE WHOLE SELF

Carl Jung described the unconscious as "the only accessible source of religious experience," and by *religious*, he meant our uniquely personal relationship with and experience of what we hold sacred in our lives.[1] In a large survey conducted on core human values, over 80 percent of respondents reported that spirituality is a dominant motivating core value for their lives.[2]

Most people who come to me for healing and growth want to get to know themselves in a much deeper and more meaningful way. One of the firefighters who came for ketamine treatment said, "I feel so dumb. I'm forty-eight years old and I just realized I really don't know who I am. How can that happen?" He had been a firefighter for twenty-three years and was one of the most respected in his city. He came to me after finding himself breaking down after a traumatic suicide and attempted homicide call that reminded him of the worst trauma he'd experienced when he was nineteen years old. He'd never had any issues with calls in his entire career, so he was surprised and very concerned to be so unsettled by this call. In our search for what might be a core issue, we discovered that he had given so much of his attention to his family, his engine and truck companies, and the community that he had completely neglected to focus on himself (a very common experience for first responders). When I asked if he allowed himself to receive, he broke into tears, realizing in that moment that he only gave and never asked for anything, which left him feeling exhausted and alone in his suffering. He desperately wanted peace, and for this to happen, he had to learn to include himself, with all the emotions, pains, traumas, and wounds he had been numbing with heavy drinking, in his own service.

Those of us who are suffering often feel disconnected or hide from ourselves because we struggle to tolerate the wounds and pain. We come to therapy hoping not only to feel better but also to create a healthy, loving relationship to the very person we are, the one we often avoid by numbing with any number of negative coping strategies, including giving too much of ourselves to others. In psychedelic psychotherapy, we learn to face ourselves and to have compassion for, tend, and eventually love ourselves deeply. Creating a holistic relationship with the whole self therefore must include discovering the hidden treasures of the unconscious—and most of this information comes in symbols, signs, metaphors, archetypes, and images.

In our daily life we have access to much of this information, but we rarely pay attention. With all our responsibilities, duties, roles, avoidance strategies like scrolling, obligations, and daily stressors, it makes sense at first why so many of us struggle to connect to ourselves, let alone pay attention to these seemingly random bits of information that surface in the mind. Yet to really know and develop a deeper relationship with ourselves, this is something we must do, and it takes slowing down and paying attention to see the signs.

How many of us miss the signs of a change coming? How many miss golden opportunities to follow our dreams or even realize when a life dream is being presented? These usually arise in signs and symbols that we overlook, ignore, or deny. Pay attention and follow those signs.

SYMBOLS AND RAVEN LEAD THE WAY

In his mid-fifties, Tim came to therapy to address a "crushing loneliness and feelings of having no direction in my life." He reported feeling numb toward everything and no emotional or physical connection with his wife.

Images of ravens seemed to come to Tim throughout his sessions. At first, he ignored them, then became interested as the images persisted. In the second session, he remembered a time he was lost in the woods as a child and feeling tremendous terror. He had run away from home a few weeks after his father died, angry with his mother for falling into a "drunken stupor and completely forgetting about me. We lived in very poor circumstances in a rural community, and no one seemed to care about how I dealt with the loss. So I ran into the forest where I always felt safe." However, as night fell he became lost and terrified.

Tim heard the caw of a raven cutting through the thick silence of his fear and grief. The raven jumped from branch to branch until it landed on one above his head. It flew to a nearby tree and cawed again. Tim had a sense to follow the bird, and as he started walking toward it, the raven flew to another tree and cawed. They did this together, the raven moving and calling for Tim to follow, until they reached a clearing that he recognized. From there, he was able to make his way home. All this came back to him in session, along with recognizing his untended grief and the anger and wild terror he carried.

His mother had not noticed he was gone.

And the terror he experienced that day never truly left him.

This memory of the raven reminded him that he was never truly alone, and despite not being cared for by his mother during that period, there always remained in him a sense of reverence, awe, and deep connection to nature. During his third session, we processed the tremendous grief he was not able to feel during his childhood and his resentment of his mother for not being present for him the way he desperately needed. He was surprised to be working on these issues because he thought he was "over it," which is a common response I hear. He realized he avoided intimacy in relationships for fear of being abandoned and chose instead to isolate himself in the very relationships in which he yearned to be held, seen, and nurtured.

In this session, we also reconnected him to his inner raven, which he could access to guide him back to his own heart whenever he felt scared and leaned toward shutting down. He shared all this with his wife as a way to begin being vulnerable with her and as a way to reconnect with her. He was building trust that she could tolerate his emotions as he was learning to access them. In the integration session, he told me that they had made love for the first time in years, and he put photos of ravens up in his home as a reminder of his journey through the dark forest.

In psychedelic psychotherapy, we take note of what arises in session. Images that may be missed or discounted in daily life can dominate a session, and that's where we can explore their meaning and connection to ourselves and our healing intentions. In addition to signs, images, symbols, and metaphors, archetypes arise from within to help us discover unexplored regions of who we are.

A CASE FOR ARCHETYPES

Archetypes offer us a way to organize how we think of ourselves and our roles in this life. Various components of our innate personality arise in the course of a session, and it helps to understand what is being made visible. Essentially, archetypes are reoccurring personality patterns and characterological motifs that can be identified across cultures and time periods. They are both very personal to who we are and universal across humanity, so they give us a deeper understanding of the way we operate and why, as well as connect us to our human community. I work with both levels, the personal and the universal, in psychedelic therapy.

Archetypes are a bridge to the invisible world that connects all people. They connect us to each other across countries, continents, and centuries. They can be found in paintings and the literary dramas of the world. These archetypes point to an interconnected human community living under the destructive forces of racism, bigotry, and brutal and false politics.

One of my favorite books that details the challenging journey toward authenticity and of honoring one's inner archetype is Madeline Miller's *Circe*. I often recommend this book, especially to my women clients who are breaking the social and cultural binds that constrain them and fully becoming themselves; however, we can all benefit from witnessing Circe's struggles and heroism while following her own path, regardless of the costs. Though her archetype is specific to healer and herbalist, her struggles are universal and thus relatable to us all.

In psychedelic psychotherapy, these motifs or character patterns become exposed in our awareness, and confusing life experiences begin to make more sense. Things that underlie our conscious awareness about ourselves come through and become clearer: why we may be driven in some ways and not others; why we long for certain types of people; why we feel compelled to do something specific out of context of our "normal" life.

Use your journal as a place to reflect, and consider these questions:

- Do you enjoy your work, truly? Can you picture what you would rather be doing, something that would fill you with purpose and energy?
- Take a moment to imagine your most fulfilling career, what you believe you were meant to do in this lifetime.
- See what comes up for you.
- Savor what you see, and notice what you feel.

This image comes from somewhere in you that is deep but waiting to emerge. We deny these images because it would mean making a *huge* change in our lives: standing up for ourselves, saying no when we mean no, saying hell yes to things that really matter, and letting other things go; setting firm boundaries; giving up toxic behaviors that make us feel good in the moment; leaving relationships that no longer serve us. Any of this sound familiar? Exploring these archetypes is worth it. Every bit of what I just wrote and more is necessary but totally worth it. The rewards for following your true archetypal energy or your most authentic self are the treasure sought in all myths.

EMBODYING THE LOST ART OF PLAY AND SEXUALITY

One of my clients is a South American woman in her sixties, a playwright known for her fierce commentary on social and gender inequalities. She survived tremendous ordeals as a child and later became paralyzed for seven years of her life. During her childhood, her mother abandoned her to escape the violence in the home, which left her to bear the wrath of her father, who began putting a gun to her head when she was fourteen and threatening her whenever he deemed it necessary. This persisted until she could escape him to a life of "self-exile" in Europe, then North America. After forty-seven years, she went back to the country of her birth looking to "return home" but found herself lost in the streets of her youth. Through our work together, she realized that her journey "from exile to home," as she phrased it, would remain incomplete until she integrated all the banished archetypes within her.

Because she was already familiar with archetypes, we dived deep into which parts of her she banished and why. She immediately identified two aspects of herself that she exiled to protect herself from men and from the pain of losing her childhood: her sexuality and her playfulness. She had been the sexual target of many men who tried to exploit her vulnerabilities for their own purposes, so she hid that goddess quality deep behind walls of steel and fire. And having her childhood taken from her at gunpoint destroyed any chance she had to be innocent and playful. Without these qualities, she felt depressed, ashamed, and rageful, and her soul was paralyzed, as her body later became.

During our prep sessions, I asked her to identify which archetypes representing sexuality and playfulness inspired her. She came back with a full list from cultures around the world. Then I encouraged her during a session to practice being like them, to feel those qualities arise within herself. Her goal was to live a life unconstricted by fear, unbound by the oppressive chains of her traumas, and to live fully embodied.

Here is the list of archetypes she found and shared with me:

> Paedia (Greek)—goddess of play and amusement (one of Aphrodite's attendants)
>
> Euphrosyne (Greek)—"merriment" (one of the Three Graces); created to fill the world with pleasant moments and goodwill
>
> Bastet (Egyptian)—"feast of drunkenness"; music, song, dance, wine; worshipped by more than seven hundred thousand people every year; represented as a cat-headed woman; originally was a fierce lioness warrior goddess of the sun
>
> Laetitia (Roman)—goddess of happiness, gladness, gaiety, luck, celebration
>
> Sunu (Chinese)—goddess of music and sex; harp player and singer
>
> Uzume (Japanese)—Shinto goddess of dance and revelry, of merry-making and humor; considered the originator of the performing arts; known as the "Heavenly Alarming Female"
>
> Dionysus (Greek)—god of festivals, play, wine, sex
>
> Eshu (Nigerian)—trickster god; messenger between heaven and earth; plays tricks on Ifa, the chief god
>
> Ishtar—goddess of sexual potency, freedom, fearlessness
>
> Chang O—goddess of the moon, banished for seeking enlightenment
>
> Saraswati—Hindu goddess of sacred art; essence of one's self; sacred authenticity

In our prep work, we spent more than six months learning to identify parts of her that she denied or repressed. She engaged in activities that helped her embody the sought-out qualities she was missing. This work alone was as powerful as any medicine journey I had witnessed. She became confident and more emboldened not only in her life but also in her artwork. And though she still deals with PTSD symptoms, they arise much less frequently and at a lower volume.

She continues to practice these "new" ways of being and reports feeling so much lighter, at ease, playful, sexual, and expressive. Her creativity now explodes in delight and flows from her like a fountain of inexhaustible pleasure. You may think this is hyperbolic, but just wait until you see what she is creating!

This is a powerful demonstration of how we can use archetypes to help us understand what is missing from the greater picture of who we are and which qualities we want to embody moving forward. Though just a small part of my work, archetypes connect us to what has been lost in the mythmaking of our lives.

Our work in the psyche never ends because we continue to plumb the depths and find what was hidden. As we find and integrate these missing pieces of our identity into the puzzle of who we are, we have new edges on the greater picture of ourselves and our interconnectedness with the universe.

COSMOS

Consciousness and awareness of the cosmos change from day to day. Some people are more open to this relationship than others. When the bills are due, when we are dealing with sickness or medical issues, when the children are crying or needing attention, when we feel alone in a crowd or feel disconnected from ourselves or our place in the world, what use is it of being aware of the greater cosmos? Will this awareness of the universe mend our broken hearts, repair relationships, make our employers treat us better, reduce racism and hatred across the globe, and reverse global warming?

No.

Psychedelic therapy does not cure and is not a panacea for every ailment we have, and the medicines alone cannot correct humanity's hardest problems. But we will.

It is my firm belief, from what I have seen in this work, that once we each have an inner shift in consciousness that changes our perspective on the importance of extending our care, concern, and actions toward the betterment of all humanity, the animals, and the planet itself, the changes we hope for will take place. These medicines are powerful, though, and certainly do have significant effects on our well-being and our sense of belonging to the greater universe in which we live and are a part.

The truth is that experiences of cosmic consciousness arise in session. Everything we see and experience on a journey exists within us and is held in our expanded awareness. We truly do contain multitudes. When we expand to the point of containing the whole universe, we know we fundamentally cannot be alone. We belong. We are a part of the whole, and we take that with us into our waking lives. Medicine experiences point directly to our interdependence and interconnectedness with all life. And we get the direct felt experience of belonging to the whole, which actually does shift our feelings of loneliness and despair. But what does it mean for our own healing and growth to be connected to this cosmic consciousness?

There is no denying that during psychedelic psychotherapy our personal identity expands to include our ancestral lineage, our environment, the larger human community, the earth, cold and empty space, and the billions of planets, stars, and galaxies that share our same matter and molecules. We find all this is conscious and alive, radiant and pulsing. That is cosmic consciousness. And this consciousness is contained within our own cells.

How is this perception shift of our expanded sense of self therapeutic? How can it help address those questions posed above? Does touching and becoming the cosmos alleviate our suffering?

The woman who explored her archetypes commented, "There is power in disidentifying from personal history because it allows me to imagine being free, to feel what it's like to be free. Touching the cosmos expands my identity to include more than just my history. It's very healing. It's very valuable when trauma embraces me. It [the cosmos] provides a safe haven. It provides a space in which I can reinvent myself in a way I want rather than how I was conditioned to be." I couldn't have said it better myself.

In a therapy that is about both us and everything, we can explore how we have become stuck in the very constricting and isolating experience of "me," with all the aches and pains, traumas, sorrows, missteps and misdeeds, and heartbreaks. So many of us become overly attached to and hyper-focused on our pain and who we think we are. Many clients come to me desperately seeking peace, space, and freedom from the very heartaches they are obsessed with. Taking the both/and cosmic approach is healing, and ultimately liberating, because we unbind from our attachment to our ego and our suffering since we learn we are fundamentally so much more.

When the cosmos presents itself in therapy, it offers the client an opportunity to discover who they truly are way beyond and deeper than the limited boundaries of their perceived self. When the client sees themselves within or as trees, dirt, insects, rivers, lava, they develop an awareness of their connection to the world around them that carries forward after the session.

When we discover we are fundamentally a part of nature and the cosmos and learn we are inextricably and undeniably connected to every human being on earth, we start to care more. It's that simple. Psychedelic psychotherapy seems to not only help us heal from our individual traumas and wounds but also increases our compassion and concern for the welfare of life itself in its inexhaustible forms.

We are at once separate, unique individuals and part of the whole, like a drop of ocean water is still the ocean in the shape of a drop. Bill

Richards writes clearly on this paradox in *Sacred Knowledge*, and it is also a central theme of Huston Smith's work, both of whom are pioneers in the field of experiential religious experiences. These concepts become therapeutically important when my clients discover and make meaning of this paradox for themselves during sessions.

THE FACE OF GOD: EVERYTHING ALL AT ONCE

It is no small thing to behold the unlimited vastness of creation. And this can be true for many during the psychedelic state; so we approach with reverence, humility, and care. And for the sake of healing, we also approach with curiosity to better understand why we are being shown what is shared.

The mysteries appear in images, shapes, feelings, signs, sounds, tastes, and more, as in a strange fever dream. Swells of emotions, bursting stars, shapeless forms standing on asteroids, flowing lava under the earth's crust, and bubbles rising out of coral, all moving and shifting to some unearthly melody deep within.

All this is you. You are all this.

What revealed secrets are these? Where does the brain create, or store, these images? Are they produced there or are they downloaded from somewhere else and projected through us?

These scenes excite, enliven, plague, perplex, frighten, and inspire us. "How is this all in me?" a client asked in awe. "I've never seen anything like this in my life. I couldn't even imagine it! What does it all mean?!"

When this happens in session (and it often does, regardless of the medication), we investigate and spend time reflecting on the montage of images and scenes, sometimes finding personal meaning relevant to their life and treatment goals, and other times resigning not to know, for now—because meaning may make itself known later or in another session.

I encourage my clients to talk to their ancestors, to allow the smells and feelings of those primal or cosmic places to overtake them so they have access to the deeper parts of the psyche needed to work through personal and ancestral issues. In psychedelic psychotherapy, the myths of our humanity find space on the wider screen of our expanded consciousness, which is usually constricted by the ego's stranglehold on our soul's imagination.

When encountering the cosmos in a session, we begin to realize we are as vast as the cosmos itself, and this knowing unlocks our ability to expand beyond our constricted sense of self. It also unlocks our potential, passions, gifts, and genius, which are often hidden beneath layers of trauma and personality patches. So many of us wear patches that limit us:

> You are this. You are that. You need to do this; you can't do that. Earn a living, don't play around with your life. Think this. Believe that. I don't have time. I'm too much. I'm not enough.

So restricting! So limiting!

As one of my clients realized, "The universe doesn't care how you load the dishwasher," which was given in response to him learning to let go of the incessant need to control others' behaviors to feel better about himself.

The cosmos is unlimited, and so are we. If you knew for sure your potential and nature were unlimited, how would life be different for you? What would you pursue? Let go of?

Most often, it takes a shakeup of your default way of thinking about and perceiving yourself and the world around you. Psychedelics can provide this, and psychedelic psychotherapy is the best method for using what arises in session as a catalyst for this deeper change.

The way to embrace the vastness of the cosmos is actually quite simple:

> Be quiet.
> Be humble.
> Be present.
> Listen.
> Observe.
> Surrender.
> Hold on to nothing.
> Be open to everything.

The presence of the cosmos can be breathtaking. When there is no fight, when we fully allow ourselves to surrender to the experience, we can experience the deep awe and wonder that so often accompany being in the presence of the great mystery of life, such as when we stand on jagged cliffs overlooking the vastness of the ocean, balance on a canyon's edge and peer down into the depths, or lie on the cool earth and stargaze on a clear night in the mountains. When we are still and quiet, the wisdom and grandeur of the universe open to us and we know for certain that we are a part of something beautiful and profound, and that we belong. This drastically helps us feel better. We don't feel so alone and isolated, and we see our own issues in a larger context, which gives us space from our suffering and adds a colorful joy to a once dreary landscape.

Exploring the psyche and cosmos in therapy is not superfluous. Doing so makes sense of and eases our suffering while promoting greater health and sense of belonging. Psychedelic psychotherapy is a gift that continues to give well beyond its conclusion.

CHAPTER 9

ORDINARY MYSTICISM

THE POWER OF
THE PRESENT MOMENT

I am writing this on a plane flying home after leading a retreat for the Sabot Foundation with special operations veterans in an undisclosed location. For me, there is nothing more inspiring and fulfilling than working with and witnessing a group of warriors, all male in this case, as their hearts crack open.

Most of their wounds do not come from the battlefield but from their childhood, when they learned early on to put on their armor and carry weapons of anger, hurt, and distrust. Their military training and experiences in combat only reinforced these defensive skills. Sometimes feelings escape, but there is nothing like alcohol to depress and numb those "fucking inefficient emotions." It's hard to be fully human, feel joy, thrive, and relate to others this way. (First responders struggle with these same issues.)

The retreat provided a safe space for the veterans to recognize the signs of this armor and learn to lay down their weapons and doff their uniforms. At the very end of this powerfully transformational retreat, I said, "You are all dismissed from duty now, forever, if you'd like," and several men wept, having let down their guard and opened their hearts.

The combination of the medicines, both psilocybin and 5-MeO-DMT, the safe container of the therapeutic space, the veterans' prep work, the loving support and psychotherapeutic stance of the staff, and the veterans' courage and willingness to engage in what they described as "harder than combat" made a profound impact on the men.

They realized how their whole lives were built around keeping their guard up, not only for others they distrusted but for themselves and their own pain. One Army veteran said feeling his sadness, fear, and grief for his years of anger and disconnection from himself was harder to sit with than being a breacher and being exposed to close-range blasts.

I often hear this from firefighters as well, that running into a burning building is easier than exploring their psyche and sitting with their feelings. Psychedelic psychotherapy often opens awareness to the emotions connected to the scenes, memories, and images of the difficult and painful parts of their youth. This is exactly what so many veterans and first responders have been repressing most of their lives under their dedicated service to others, mental toughness, emotional invulnerability, attempts to control external circumstances and people, and substance and alcohol use. The cost of their service to their emotional, physical, and psychological lives is huge, and this type of therapy uncovers all of it.

One retreatant, a former Marine who has worked as a defense contractor for ten years after his decade of service, deployed a combined total of fifty times! His bravery in coming to a retreat to unlock and face the inner cost of decades of combat and contracting experience is greater than what it takes for him to return downrange, where he is more comfortable. This became very apparent during his time on the medicines. The mushrooms and the 5-MeO-DMT made it very apparent how the darkness of war and defense contracting consumed him. He could see nothing but death and darkness, all unprocessed. During his psilocybin journey, he even became suspicious of us, imagining that we "were out to get" him, which was only dispelled because we were so loving and tender with him. It was no wonder he spent his time between deployments drinking heavily and isolating, waiting to return to his tribe, who understands and accepts him as he engages in work he feels born for.

He was willing but ultimately unable at that time to face the deeper pain of his life that drove him to isolation and alcohol. Acknowledging his truth and accepting just where he was, combined with setting intentions for inner peace and learning whether there is a higher power, were the first steps on his road to healing.

The last day of the retreat, I gathered the group for one more exercise. After a grounding practice, I played the Wood Brothers' "Heart Is the Hero" while they sat and listened to the lyrics that so accurately describe some of the process they went through during the retreat. I then invited the men to write a love letter to themselves. With full permission to share, here are some of the letters these courageous warriors wrote to themselves and shared in the closing circle:

> Letter to B,
> I must say that I am surprised that it has taken nearly seventy years to come to love the man that B has always been. While I have always liked who I am, I have never gotten close enough to myself to fall in love.
>
> As a result, I have missed out on so much compassion, joy, and happiness that could otherwise have been.
>
> But now, in this seventieth year, I have been blessed to be introduced to a heavenly group of people that helped me find new purpose for the autumn of my life. I intend to go back

to work utilizing my creative skills and I know that it will not only serve others but will unlock my mind and soul and restore the joy that has been missing for the last few years. Thanks for doing this, B.
I love you!

Dear C,
I am sorry for treating you so poorly over the years. I am grateful of the recognition and awareness that I no longer have to punish myself to survive. I am grieving this right now. I can love myself and start being aware of the self-hatred and self-sabotage that has led you to think that you don't deserve to be treated well with love and compassion.

I love you, and I'm sorry. As you move forward, recognize that there's grace when you fall short, and unconditional love. It's okay to grieve and it's okay to love yourself. May God lead you every day, and receive the grace that God has given you. Take this and give to others as God guides you.

G,
What a journey. You have lived, loved, fought, and made countless mistakes. Although in the past you have judged these mistakes as if you were a Creator. I have found these amazing people who have changed me. It is okay to love. It is okay to make mistakes and give yourself grace. I always enjoyed how you constantly challenged yourself to push beyond what was thought possible. You live life like anything is possible and after the journey this weekend you have realized it is okay to love yourself. I love you, my friend.

As you continue your journey remember the shit that has happened to you doesn't define you. Instead, your heart defines who you are. Continue to love yourself and let your inner child run around without limits. This energy you have found is unstoppable. The love you now feel inside is to be shared with the world. Now go ahead and share this shit with everyone you encounter. Never stop being you, brother!

As the men read their letters, not a dry eye remained. These men wept for themselves. They wept for each other. They wept for their individual and collective pain. And the soothing waters of hope sprang from the sacred wells of their hearts. As we parted, the hugs were long and we looked deeply into one another's eyes. We all remain connected to this day.

This work is extraordinary and yet so simple. Underneath all the mental conditions, habits, and defenses, the hidden treasure of our deepest truths lies waiting to be discovered. These medicines often act like a sort of truth serum, dissolving the ego's defenses, allowing what needs to be seen, felt, and spoken to arise for the sake of healing and transformation. As one client put it, "This medicine allows me to move out of the way and experience and exposes my internal reality without any distortion. It just comes through. What I need most is right here."

I couldn't have said that any better.

After retreats, many of the veterans text photos to our group and to me personally of the simple things that now have more meaning. Retreats leave them feeling connected, in awe and wonder. Sunsets, sunrises, leaves on water, snow falling on red mailboxes, light hitting windows of tall city buildings, a baby's smiling face. These simple moments, which are now felt to be profound, become gifts in their healing and thriving. Psychedelic psychotherapy first transformed their perception of themselves, and then their perception of the world. And through these ordinary mystical moments during normal waking life, they become warriors in the garden.

This is true for most of my clients who, through this therapy, have reconnected to the simple beauty of life and to their own soul.

A THERAPY OF RECONNECTION

This work teaches us to slow down and enjoy this life we've been gifted. As difficult as it can be, with as many untended wounds as we have, and because the loads we carry are heavy, it is still a precious gift to be alive. To taste your favorite food, drink cool water, hold the hand of your lover. This is the time to relish what we can of this life.

Being grateful for the present moment and not taking our life for granted, as difficult as it can be at times, are such powerful remedies for depression, anxiety, and trauma. Traumas often leave us feeling perpetually scared and unable to experience the simple joys of life, which can lead to feeling depressed. Psychedelic therapies and medicines are known for reconnecting us to the beauty of our surroundings and the blessings that we do experience in our life that we often deny. To be reconnected to the joys that the present moment brings is not arbitrary. It is essential for a life of happiness. In fact, what most of my clients express is gratitude for feeling the joy of simple pleasures returned to them.

I am sharing this as a human who knows suffering. As one who had an emotionally and psychologically tormented upbringing, who lived under the terrorizing shadow of the Holocaust, who had and worked through a drug addiction, who had and lost a beautiful marriage, who hurt others and lived in shame for it, and who struggled with suicidality and existential dread, I understand your pain. And what I know to be true, and what I am sharing in this book, is that when we dedicate ourselves to these practices, we can find the treasures buried deep in our pain. When we find the endless beauty of life as it is shown during these sessions or during a mystical experience, we can live with joy, peace, and ease, not in spite of the challenges and traumas but because of them.

We often rush through this world of vibrant colors, tastes, smells, textures, and shapes just to be done with the day. We often focus on what we dislike about our lives, ourselves, our circumstances, and other people. This makes life disagreeable, drab, dreary, gray, atonal, and uninspired. Numbing ourselves and rushing through life are the great soul crushers.

Psychedelic psychotherapy has the potential to wake us up to what we've been missing, which is the purity of life in its most simple form. This is ordinary mysticism. We can discover again that life is beautiful in its simplicity. And that it's around us and free. Humanity is consumed by new and exciting technologies, which often cost more than most people can afford, hence overspending, indebtedness, and overworking to compensate for this habit. What we are missing are the simple pleasures that life offers that often cure us. Spend an hour with your phone and register how you actually feel. Spend an hour sitting by a river and be aware of how you feel. Psychedelics and this new therapy bring the senses back to life, which is essential for our overall well-being and thriving as human beings.

Just as exploring the psyche and the cosmos are not superfluous, neither is spending time cultivating our inner mystic, the one who sees in vivid color and who is deeply connected to life, even when life is difficult and painful. Ordinary mysticism is an internal state of being that exists independently of external circumstances. Pain, aging, and our eventual death are natural factors in life. We cannot get out of them. What we can experience is deep peace, connection, belonging, awe, and wonder at the beautiful simplicity of life. And psychedelic psychotherapy can provide the conditions in which this is more likely to happen for us.

APPLIED MYSTICISM: FOR THE BOYS IN BROOKLYN

In the spring of 2024, I had a conversation with Steve Stein, founder of BetterListen!, at a summit called "Psychedelics, Therapy, and Society." He and Jon Kabat-Zin had created a podcast called *StreetSmart Wisdom* to bring ancient wisdom traditions to "the street level."

He talked about growing up in Brooklyn and thinking about how he would introduce or share the profound teachings of ancient and Indigenous traditions and practices with the "boys I grew up with," who were rough-and-tumble men.

This immediately brought to mind the work I do with first responders and combat veterans, so I shared my approach for doing just that with the populations I serve. I described how I had been working with Sashi, a police officer, both in traditional and ketamine-assisted psychotherapy.

Sashi came to me to address concerns he had in his relationship. He loved his job as a police officer and on the SWAT team. He had served in two different cities during his eighteen-year career and was as close to embodying a Knight archetype as anyone I have ever met. He was dedicated to being a guardian of justice, willing to sacrifice his life to defend and protect any community members in need. He was also a dedicated husband and father but was struggling with his spouse in ways that were quite common for first responders. His daily calls included domestic violence situations, teenage suicides, fatal car accidents, overdoses and drug-related deaths, medical emergencies in the homeless population, and dealing with the many bureaucratic and administrative challenges in the police department.

Because of the extremely tense and stressful nature of his work, Sashi had, like most first responders, developed a coping strategy that included compartmentalizing the emotions evoked by the horrors and traumas of humanity. Although this makes sense to do on a call when he could not stop to weep for the death of a child, cutting off his emotions completely did not work in the family and in regular human life.

He was unaware he had been doing this, and when he received feedback that he seemed distant and not emotionally available, his response was that he was always doing his best to help his wife and solve problems. Another typical first responder response! As we continued our work together, which included him becoming aware of his internal emotional world, Sashi realized how closed off he had become and how distant he felt from himself as well. He wasn't feeling joy, ease, playfulness, or creativity either. Also, the world was a place of evil and danger to him, not one of beauty. Unfortunately, this is true for many first responders and veterans who have spent their careers immersed in the darker side of humanity.

In our first ketamine session, his heart burst wide open and he began to feel everything he had suppressed over the many years of his career, and his profound grief at the dissolution of his marriage flooded him for the first time. He experienced this over a series of sessions. These heart openings, as hard as they were, gave him greater access not only to his emotional world and hidden aspects of his psyche but also to the beauty of the world itself, which he had been closed off from because of the terrible nature of the calls he went on. His defenses softened and he *felt* love for the first time in years. His senses, which were always on alert for danger, began to sense what was pleasurable to him. He reported flavors returning when eating meals and started to enjoy songs and melodies that had lost their appeal (Sashi was a trained musician who had stopped playing once he became a cop).

After just three sessions, he was able to apply this new way of being and thinking at home and at work. Although his marriage continued to dissolve, he no longer closed himself off from his emotions and eventually learned to act in a more open-hearted way toward those he served in the community and even those he arrested.

Fast-forward...

Two years later, Sashi was on my couch and said he had a fantasy during his morning meditation: He had imagined a perpetrator attacking him. While he saw himself grappling with the man, he heard himself say, "I love this person, he is just like me. I can use force without anger, subduing him with compassion." He then told me, "I no longer want to hurt anybody, just stop them."

And just as I was wrapping up this chapter, Sashi texted me:

> I have been feeling the nauseating gut punch of primal sorrow the last couple of days. It feels like it's all related to not living with my son full-time, but there's more to it than that. During my fifteen-minute meditation time this evening, I spent thirteen or fourteen minutes of it crying like a baby. At one point, I pictured myself holding and comforting him. He slowly morphed into me as a child and I realized I was holding and comforting me as a boy. I am committed to facing this head-on and not hurting myself or anyone else by acting out because I am avoiding the issue. I will wield the fierce sword of compassion.

I am not making this up. This is a true story.

The power of the present moment. Being present with what *is* often brings the very healing we need for the suffering we face. And though the present moment brings challenges and difficulties, it contains the beauty, awe, majesty, and love we need to truly enjoy our lives.

And for no one is this more true than for those who are dying.

GLIOBLASTOMA AND LOVING WHAT IS HERE

For most of us, facing our mortality brings up immense fear and deep aversion. The simplest truth of our existence is that we, and all things, die. It's nature, and it's natural. But so many in their fear of this natural occurrence spend their lives avoiding what could be a potent practice for thriving. The saying inscribed on the back of the wooden block struck with a mallet by Zen monks to announce meditation time is this:

> Be aware of the great matter of birth and death.
> Life passes swiftly.
> Wake up! Wake up!
> Do not waste this life!

We do not know when or how, but we will die, and accepting this fact can help us live our life to the fullest. We can spend more of our attention and energy on things that matter. For Maria, life was coming to an end. She was in her late forties with two teenagers and had a glioblastoma, an incurable brain tumor. She came to me to find peace with her death, knowing she was leaving behind two children and her husband.

She carried great guilt about leaving her children and feared they would not be taken care of the way she wanted. Her husband and she had vastly different parenting styles. Would her children have a balanced upbringing? What would they do without her?

Her goals were to make peace with her life, forgive herself for past mistakes, and accept and allow her husband to just be himself. She wanted to stop judging him for how different he was from her. She wanted to let go and trust, basically, to give up control, which she loved holding on to. She loved directing things. But here was death, and she could not direct it.

Our prep sessions were tailored to move her closer to these goals before the journey, to help her let go of rigidity, the need to control herself and others. She truly seemed accepting of her death, but trusting others was so difficult. And with this rigidity came tiresome stress and, at times, a joylessness. She loved to argue, with herself and with life.

And this was so apparent as she began her journey. She spent the first half of the session arguing with characters in her life who would appear to her. She had gripes. She had complaints. I asked her if this was how she lived, and she said it was. I asked if she wanted to be different. She did. She wanted to feel peace and ease and joy. I wondered aloud what gratitude would feel like, how it might help her reorganize how she saw her life and maybe allow her peace in the final months of it. I asked if she could soften and express her deeper feelings about her life.

Her life began to show itself to her more rapidly. A best friend, her children's births, the great love affair of her life with her husband. Her regrets and remorse. Her joys and challenges. Her heart opened to her, her body, her breath, heartbeat, tingling skin. She felt love for life and saw how beautiful it was in its simplicity. She loved her children deeply and felt a sense of trust for their well-being arise. She saw her husband in his uniqueness and loved him for it more than ever. She felt trust for him, that he would be the wonderful father their children needed. She wept and laughed and finally quieted into the silence of awe that most mystics know in the face of a sunset.

She came out resolved to spend as much time with her family as possible, just being. Just living was enough for her. Whatever time she had left would be spent loving life and her family, despite whatever the cancer would bring. She didn't want to control anything, force anything, judge anything. Why waste any of her precious time? This was her hope and her commitment.

She died three months later.

Ordinary mysticism is not just for "spiritual" people. It is for the "Boys in Brooklyn," first responders and veterans, parents, those leading ordinary lives, and those facing death. The beauty of the present moment is available to all of us, in all moments of our lives, and gives us access to the unconditional love that we long for and that is necessary to heal and thrive. The more we touch it, the greater our sense of joy, belonging, and care for ourselves, others, and the world in which we live becomes. And it is a tonic for our suffering.

Try it for yourself. You don't need psychedelic psychotherapy. Just for today, *slow down* and *notice* what is alive within and around you.

Literally stop and smell the roses. See what the present moment has to offer you. Listen for birdsong, watch leaves moving in the wind, enjoy your favorite song without distraction, feel your own breath and heartbeat. Experience what sages throughout time have tried to teach us: Ordinary life can be spectacular and extraordinary in its simplicity. I can almost guarantee you won't be disappointed and will feel better for it.

PART THREE

THE HEART IS HOME

The sweetness and delights of the resting-place are in proportion to the pain endured on the Journey. Only when you suffer the pangs and tribulations of exile will you truly enjoy your homecoming.

—Rumi

CHAPTER 10

INTEGRATION
THE ART OF CURATING THE GOOD LIFE

Matt is a kind and humble forty-something-year-old man from LA. He came to me wanting to elevate his life. Although there was nothing really "wrong"—he was happily married, had a good career in the medical supply field, and had great friends—something was lacking and something "felt off."

When he would start to explore new ideas or lean toward having new experiences, he would freeze and remain committed to what he was already doing. Fear: the mind killer, as Frank Herbert wrote in *Dune*. In Matt's case, fear: freedom and fun killer. But where and when was his fear born?

This is quite a common theme for many clients in their forties and fifties who come for therapy to enhance their lives. This is what my transformational coaching program is about, which often uses ketamine-assisted psychotherapy to help clients find and heal the constrictions that keep them from thriving. But so many are stuck in the familiar and attached to the comfort of the known.

My work is not always about healing trauma but also about discovering what is most alive within a client, and then encouraging them to live out what is found within. And Matt longed to experience true freedom, to express his deepest self and let it out to play. So we had to find the original story of his fear.

During an integration coaching session, which occurred after his sessions with the medicine, he recalled a previous journey in which he explored what he thought were images and experiences from potential previous lives. He said he felt so free during his journey into his past lives, where he expressed himself, his sexuality, his gifts without shame or fear of punishment.

During his journey, he flashed forward to a memory in his living room when he was thirteen. He had not yet come out as gay, but he suspected his mother knew. He remembers her sharing news articles about gay men dying alone from AIDS. He remembers feeling confused, frightened, and ashamed. In his journey, he became that thirteen-year-old, alienated, alone, and afraid. This thing he knew to be true about himself, did it lead to a lonely death? Is that what his mother wanted him to know? What he remembers is knowing that being himself was not safe.

In our discussion, he said these feelings continued into his early twenties when everyone was still very afraid of HIV/AIDS, and he lived with uncertainty. For much of his life, he felt stifled and had difficulty expressing himself. What he wanted most was to fully be himself, but he would freeze instead. This was true of how he operated in the world, in his job, in relationships. But now he was ready to integrate what he learned about himself in that journey and in our integration sessions into his life. He was ready to take flight in a life of authenticity and freedom. And enjoy himself in the process. "At first, getting to know myself was really uncomfortable, like I was doing something wrong. But then I realized it could be enjoyable to get to know me. It doesn't have to be so serious!"

I totally agree. I know it's scary to redefine ourselves against the conditioning, expectations, and old patterns. But we might discover we actually *like* ourselves! Just as we are.

Can you imagine that? Actually enjoying your own company? I'm serious. Part of my duty, in sessions and certainly in the integration phase, is to help clients fall in love with the person they are by really learning about themselves and curating a good life that is specific to who they are.

An essential step in the psychedelic psychotherapeutic process, integration is when we incorporate our insights and new understandings into our daily life. Whereas the psychedelic experience and the therapeutic sessions are helpful, healing, and transformational in themselves, the lessons must be turned into daily practices and behaviors to concretize the changes we are making.

The truth is, the really hard part of this whole process is going home and facing the parts of our lives that were created out of the trauma, resentment, anxiety, and depression we were seeking to work through and heal. Old habits and old feelings continuously surface because these conditions take time to dissolve within the newfound spaciousness and loving awareness that we built during therapy. And what are some of the best ways to relate to ourselves as we build new behaviors while experiencing the old ones?

Grace
Patience
Understanding
Compassion

These are not merely words or concepts; they are practices we incorporate into our daily life.

Occasionally, our experiences are powerful enough to disrupt our normal patterns and habits of being: think accidents, near-death experiences, divorce, the death of a loved one, transcendental moments of oneness. These can be shocking to the core, changing our worldview in a moment. Some psychedelic experiences can be like this too. However, in general, most sustained and long-term changes need intentional, attention-setting repetition and reinforcement to become a new worldview or behavior.

The integration process is focused on creating and committing to practical and reasonable changes in behavior, perception, and thinking in our daily life. We are not looking for huge shifts because they are difficult to sustain. We want to focus on small, realistic changes.

I encourage my clients to be aware of the small, subtle shifts they perceive after our therapeutic sessions. I was working with Amanda, who sought psychedelic psychotherapy to rediscover the peace and freedom she felt while living abroad before settling down in a marriage and having children. During an integration session, she was talking about a situation with her kids that would have normally driven her mad. "I wanted to yell at my kids, but I didn't." When I asked what happened, she responded, "I felt myself becoming angry. I heard what I was about to yell in my mind, and then I decided to take some deep breaths and to calmly talk to my kids about what was happening and what I needed from them. This seems like a small thing, maybe, but it is so important for me. I don't want to yell at them. They become scared of me. I want to work with them and be kind. I never got that as a child. I felt so much calmer doing it this way and was able to actually enjoy the rest of my morning." She discovered how to be mindful, calm herself down, and keep her values in the forefront. She was integrating what she learned in our sessions in her life at home.

During the integration process, we choose which behaviors we want to practice. We determine which to practice by becoming aware of our values and our overall health and wellness goals. When we have clarity around our values and goals, it becomes easier to choose new behaviors over the habituated behaviors that no longer serve us.

THE HARD SIDE

To be clear, the journey can remain difficult during the integration phase. Contracting back into ourselves, our old ways of being, is quite common. Contracting after expansion is natural, just as some flowers open in the day and close at night. No one can stay expanded all the time, so we must learn to be tolerant of and compassionate toward contracting or retracting states of mind and energy after psychedelic experiences. This is why having a good support system in place is essential. Who can you call? The integration phase lays out a map of support that includes trusted friends and community, a therapist, a mentor, and an integration support group.

People often struggle to return to their normal routines, ones that were created out of stress rather than health-oriented thinking. I've heard clients complain that their spouses or partners seem distant or stuck in the past, while they are moving into a new future. Most often, clients feel more depressed than before. But in most of these cases, it's just that they are much more aware of their historical emotional baseline. All this can be anticipated and worked with.

Underlying and repressed emotions may surface. "It was like the Hulk came out!" It can look ugly sometimes. In very rare cases, clients report feeling dissociated and disembodied for weeks or months afterward. They just couldn't ground themselves back in their body and daily life. They remain disoriented or have a sense of dislocation. But as far as I am aware, in all the years I have been working in this field, none of my clients have reported long-lasting distress after their psychedelic experience. Some clients might experience manic-like symptoms or feel unsure of who they are. One client, a healthy male in his early forties, reported feeling an elevation in energy with heightened pleasant mood for four days after he took 5-MeO-DMT on retreat in Mexico. Again, though these longer-lasting effects are rare in my experience, it's important to know that they are a possibility.

At this time, we do not have enough data to suggest who may be likely to experience prolonged effects. I am not writing this to scare you away from psychedelic psychotherapy but to make you aware. If this is an issue or concern for you, you should talk with your therapist and seek support from those who are trained in issues of spiritual emergence and emergencies.

We can never predict the outcomes of this type of therapy or of psychedelics in general, so it's wise to seek counsel from those who are trained. It is your responsibility to protect and educate yourself before engaging in any activity where there is risk, especially psychedelics. Three good books that explore these topics are Jack Kornfield's *After the Ecstasy, the Laundry: How the Heart Grows Wise on the Spiritual Path*; Jules Evans's *Breaking Open: Finding a Way Through Spiritual Emergency*; and Stan Grof and Christina Grof's *Spiritual Emergency: When Personal Transformation Becomes a Crisis*.

A good integration plan starts during the preparation phase with solid education and aftercare planning. It is the responsibility of the therapist to offer this and of the client to ask for it. The better the preparation, the smoother the integration can be. Assuming this has been done, what does a good integration plan look like?

THE ART OF CURATING

Once we get through the therapeutic sessions, the client and I establish our integration plan, which will include specific daily practices such as mindfulness, prayer, exercise, and mindful communication skills. We choose which new behaviors and people the client wants to include in their life. We begin to curate their lifestyle activities and new habits derived from the learning and growth experienced during the psychedelic sessions. The client learns to choose consciously and more carefully who they want to spend time with, which activities to engage in, what to do for a living, and how to talk to their loved ones and those they have conflicts with. Each piece of their life can be chosen with care because their future well-being depends on the choices they make now.

Think of yourself like a jigsaw puzzle with missing pieces and no edges. You discover some of what's missing in psychedelic psychotherapy but no edges, because you learned you are boundless like the cosmos and will forever expand your understanding of yourself. Integration is adding pieces to the puzzle that is you, and the model I use is a three-step process: reflection, building, and practicing.

Reflection

The first phase of integration begins between medicine sessions if there are multiple sessions or at the end of the single medicine session. During our work, I ask my clients to journal new insights about themselves; shifts in mood, cognition, and beliefs they become aware of; and changes in behaviors and to document their experiences of trying new behaviors. Trying a new behavior means actively practicing a new way of acting and being aware of the impact on their mood, mindset, body, and relationships. Reflection is ongoing through the entire psychotherapeutic process, but we spend time specifically going over their reflections at the beginning of the integration process.

Following are examples of reflection prompts I use. Clients only write on those that pertain to them and their specific therapy goals.

- What new abilities and skills have you gained?
- What new feelings are present?
- Is there any release of trauma constriction in your body and mind?
- What are your depressive, anxious, or trauma symptoms like now?
- What truths have you discovered?
- What does being authentic look and feel like now?
- What are your self-care needs and behaviors?
- Did you meet any of your therapy goals, and how do you know if you did?

- Did you meet your future self? If so, what did you see, hear, or learn? What were they doing?
- Did you meet any of your past selves or your inner child? What work did you do with them, and what is your relationship with them now?
- Any contact with ancestors? If so, what did you see, hear, or learn? What were they doing?
- What is your relationship with your body like now? Any new behaviors and attitudes toward your body?
- What changes have you made with your substance use? Any differences in how you relate to or use substances?

Reflection is a way to get to know yourself better without adding harmful layers of judgment or shame. In fact, true reflection is full of compassion and love, because it is the loving witness inside you that observes and reports back. Because there is no harsh judgment or shame about what you observe, even if you don't like or want what you see, you can utilize what you see to your benefit.

You need to see yourself in a way that doesn't cause you more pain and suffering. The very *way* you see yourself determines what comes next. If you see yourself with harsh judgment, you will shame yourself, which puts you back to where you started. If you see yourself with understanding and compassion, you offer yourself grace and can use the experience to grow. It's that simple.

Reflection is a spiritual practice.

We then take what you discovered in the reflection phase and begin building a plan to sustain your growth.

Building an Ecosystem of Support and Clarifying Your Values

This is where you get to design what looks good in the home of your life. During this phase, we curate new ways of being with your tastes, style, and values in mind. Things you genuinely like about your life stay, and things you don't like, go (reasonably). Even though this is the time in the integration process to reevaluate what no longer serves you, those of us working in the field usually strongly encourage clients *not* to make big decisions right after psychedelic experiences or therapeutic sessions.

Bad trips are nothing compared to the horror stories about people quitting their jobs or leaving their spouses immediately after a session or two. I totally understand the impulse, but doing so right then is akin to drunk texting, which is never a good idea. Even if an individual was considering these very moves before they began therapy and gained the clarity and confidence needed to move forward with these very important decisions during PP, we still recommend taking time in the integration process to mindfully and carefully curate the next phase of life. Unless there is immediate danger, there is usually no need to rush, and being skillful and conscientious will pay off in the long run. So how do we curate what comes next?

I am guided by two models during this phase: Acceptance and Commitment Therapy (ACT), and Cassandra Vieten's Ecosystem of Change. For me, the ecosystem is the big picture of the needed integrated support system, and ACT is a closer look at the individual pieces that eventually complete the ecosystem, so let's start there first.

The ACT model suggests at least these nine core human values are universal: family relations; marriage, couple, and intimate relations; parenting; friendships and social relationships; employment; recreation; spirituality; community; physical well-being. I use a worksheet to help clients assess how much they value these domains versus how much time they put into cultivating them. They say this is a very eye-opening exercise.

The discrepancies can be unsettling but inspiring. Clients often see why they feel so misaligned, depressed, or anxious in their lives. For example, they might value creativity, friendships, and recreation highly, but put no time toward those activities. No wonder our souls feel so depressed!

During the building phase, in creating a reasonable plan of practices, it is vital that clients be completely honest with themselves on this worksheet. For example, if someone grew up in a strict religious household but does not value religion or spirituality, they may, out of guilt, ascribe greater value to that domain than if they were being honest about how much they value religion. After a few psychedelic psychotherapy sessions, the impulse to lie to appease other people diminishes in favor of speaking one's truth, so doing this activity in the integration process is quite helpful. I encourage clients to speak their truths and honestly assess what they hold dear versus what can be left alone at this time in their life. When clients fill out this worksheet honestly, specific value domains of interest become obvious, and curating the pieces that matter becomes easier.

In Dr. Vieten's Ecosystem of Change, we build an integrative system that supports the continuity and sustainability of the transformational process. This new model of integration is designed to help one create changes in their life that otherwise would be difficult to do without such support. The conditions for long-lasting change are brought together into a living, thriving ecosystem that is interconnected and interdependent for the benefit of practicing new behaviors and taking on new mindsets. This becomes the ecosystem of our life: friends, community, spiritual and self-care practices, meaningful work, imagination and creativity, guidance and mental health support in the form of therapy or mentorship, and so on.

In the Ecosystem of Change model, each piece interacts with others, creating a system that is dynamic and fluid but always supportive of growth. When one element is weak or out of reach, the other pieces add strength and support. Dr. Vieten suggests that sustained positive mental health can be achieved within an integrative system that supports change and transformation. Sometimes my clients and I map out their ecosystem using large pieces of paper and art supplies. We look at the elements that are already in place and those they wish to add in support of transforming their learning into sustained ways of being.

Other clinicians, therapists, and healers will most likely use their own models of care and support during the integration process. However, I have found these two models very helpful during the building phase because they emphasize one's uniquely personal values within the context of an overall integrative, supportive system.

Curating your list of new behaviors, activities, mindsets, and practices is an art form. It takes knowing your own style, tastes, and heart's values, which may have been difficult to access before engaging in psychedelic psychotherapy but should be easier afterward. Once personal values are determined and an ecosystem is built to support the changes, it is time to turn these ideas into actions.

Practicing What Matters

The next chapter is devoted to embodiment and living deeply, and it begins with practice. On the last day of retreats, during the integration circle, I often tell retreatants, "You are gonna suck at being this new version of you. The way you feel right now will not last, but the lessons and your learning will. Be patient and graceful with yourselves as you begin to practice being this new version of you." They usually all laugh and groan.

It takes dedication, discipline, and consistency to turn practices into a lifestyle, into a way of being, where sought-out behaviors, good moods, and positive thinking happen on their own. So, what are we practicing in this stage of integration? That depends on what was discovered in reflection and which practices were chosen during the building phase. Let's take a moment to describe what a practice is.

In their book *Living Deeply: The Art and Science of Transformation*, authors Schlitz, Vieten, and Amorak define *practice* as having five components: intention, attention, repetition, guidance, and community. They settled on this definition after completing a content analysis of more than fifty interviews with world religious, spiritual, and modern integrative transformational practice leaders who had described the process of transformation from the perspective of the spiritual teachings they were grounded in. I have used this definition of *practice* ever since I started my mentorship under Cassandra Vieten many years ago and have been blessed to coteach this as a course with Cassandra for many years now.

These five components can be used in any discipline or practice:

1. *Intention* is the desired outcome, the why. What do you hope to gain from meditation, dancing, drumming, painting, running, and so forth? This becomes a guidepost or a beacon on the horizon. When we forget, when we choose something else that hurts us, when we don't want to, our intention is there to remind us of what's important.
2. *Attention* is mental focus, keeping your mind on the task at hand. The best learning happens when the mind is not distracted, when it picks up the subtleties of the experience, those little moves that make a dance or the strokes and shading that complete a painting.
3. *Repetition* creates the necessary neural pathways that lead to expertise and mastery of a practice. Pro athletes' bodies move into position before their minds tell them to. You are training your body as much as your mind when repeating patterns. So much of my work with clients in the integration phase is encouraging them to practice a new behavior regardless of the immediate results. It takes time for practices to bear fruits, so we must be patient and have grace while we repeat a new behavior.
4. *Guidance* can happen through mentorship, by being a student and taking a teacher; by speaking to a spiritual leader; by going to therapy; by having the wise counsel of trusted friends. We can't see what is in our blind spots. We need reassurance when we're scared and lost. We need

to be held accountable. We need encouragement when we want to quit. I often hear people saying, "I can do this myself," which is a very isolating fantasy. We really cannot do this by ourselves. We need support. I have an amazing therapist, two spiritual teachers, a mentor, my sister, a very kind and wise ex-wife, and a handful of very trusted friends I turn to for counsel.

5. *Community* happens when a group of people who have similar intentions gather to engage in an activity or to cocreate an experience. Buddhists call this *sangha*. Yogis call this *satsang*. This is the purpose of going to church, temple, or mosque. It's why we have funerals, weddings, bar mitzvahs, ecstatic dance events, and music festivals. This is why as humans we have participated in community sweat lodges, Sun Dances, whale hunts and celebrations, and tribal medicine ceremonies throughout our history. Engaging in an activity as part of a community with shared intentions has been shown to increase the power of that experience for all who participate. Community is a group of people who get you, who understand your lifestyle, culture, and ways of seeing and living in the world. These are people who have your back when you need support.

In this stage of integration, most clients are so ready to continue feeling the peace, ease, freedom, relief, and energy they feel immediately after the psychedelic experience. They feel that making the changes that seemed impossible before they started therapy are now in reach. It is not easy, at first, because old habits and mindsets are still present and strong, but their number and frequency have been reduced, so a client's willingness and readiness to commit to new ways of being and thinking are high.

With increased self-awareness after the experience, it becomes easier for us to spot the signs of mental distress as they arise. One retired police officer struggled with very low self-esteem ever since his father had died during his teens, which left his mother overwhelmed and doing her best to take care of four kids, leaving him lost in the shuffle. In the integration phase, he committed to using his newfound self-awareness to monitor and change his internalized self-loathing. He shared this in an integration session about his previous few weeks of practice: "I started seeing how often I was hard on myself. I can't believe I was that negative. I would say negative things for nothing, missing a small patch of lawn when mowing. I would never talk to anyone that way. Now when I hear a thought like that, I don't indulge it. I give myself space to feel what I need to and then am kinder to myself. I say to myself, 'I've got this.'" Seeing himself so clearly as a good human being worthy of his own attention and already having touched love for himself and peace in his sessions gave him the internal model he needed for this new self-love practice.

When he and I worked on turning self-love into a practice, this is what we came up with:

> *Intention:* To treat himself better, with kindness, encouragement, support, and love. He wanted to focus on himself and his dreams, which he had never done in his life.
>
> *Attention:* He trained his mind to be aware of his self-talk, to listen to its messages, and to feel his body's response. He paid attention to both his mind and his body in this practice. Negative self-talk feels terrible in the body, like being abused. He was able to monitor his negative thinking by becoming more aware of his body's reactions and feelings. Sometimes he would hear the negative thinking and then sense his body's response. This is where he put his attention.

Repetition: He chose to do this daily for a number of weeks between integration sessions. He would journal what he saw and experienced.

Guidance: He was coming to me for integrative coaching after his ketamine sessions.

Community: He joined a monthly group for first responders who were all working on these issues.

He is now starting to enjoy his retirement and is looking forward to learning more about himself and is now focusing on becoming a chaplain!

A NOTE FROM THE WISE

Old ways of being will still arise, and our job is to monitor and respond in a way that aligns with our deepest values. This in itself is a practice. We are not going for perfect. We are going for consistent.

As I began my Ayurvedic training many years ago, my teacher, Richard Haynes, encouraged me to do my practices 51 percent of the time. At first, I balked and said, "I can do these all the time!" and he quietly stared at me for what seemed like hours until I realized my inner perfectionist was bragging and way overconfident. When I really listened to what he suggested, I felt a deep sense of relief and gratitude. I finally had the grace to not have to push myself, to be more relaxed in my learning, to not be perfect. Over time that 51 percent became 80 percent naturally. And though I am no longer in training, many of these practices have simply become a way of life for me. I hear this from many of my clients who dedicate time in their day to their own well-being: New behaviors just become a way of being for them.

When Cassandra and I teach on the transformational process, we encourage participants to commit to one or two new behaviors for one or two years to get the full benefit of transforming a practice into a way of being. The usual response? People almost yell: "One to two years?! That's too long!" Our response? "How many years have you been hurting yourself with negative self-talk, indulging negative moods, clinging to outdated beliefs about yourself? You've already committed thirty to fifty years or more to those behaviors and are an expert. Imagine what two years of practicing self-love, self-compassion, patience, and grace can do for you."

I can feel your responses as you read this. "Dang, am I ready for this? I don't think I have time." Shush that part! Over time, it gets easier and smoother to do what seems impossible right now. And the benefits along the way are exponential, cumulative, and last a lifetime.

AN INTEGRATIVE STORY

All three stages of the integration process are equally important and create a model you can use anytime you are ready to make a change. Reflect, build a reasonable plan and ecosystem of support, and then practice one or two new behaviors until they become engrained and sustained in your life.

I was working with a twenty-three-year-old man who was struggling with depression, awkward social interactions, impulse control issues, angry outbursts, chronic low self-esteem, and suicidality. He was extremely bright and creative and was working hard, but struggling, to get into the film industry, which was his life's dream. He found it hard to follow through on his ideas, which contributed to his self-loathing and the idea that something must be wrong with him. He relied a lot on his parents because they lived close by and was embarrassed about this. During our prep session, I wanted to better understand his chronic depression, which he said started in third grade. He'd felt he was different from other kids but didn't know in what way. He often felt embarrassed of himself and out of place, like he didn't really belong. He struggled to communicate what he thought and often couldn't relate to others on an emotional level.

Although it was not my role to diagnose him, we did talk about the possibility that he was on the autism spectrum, and he lit up, saying he and his friends thought this was true. We talked about how neurodiversity can play out in a person's life, and he started to do his own research between our sessions.

Because of his struggle to access his emotions, I wondered how ketamine psychotherapy was going to work with or benefit him. In our sessions, we were able to build his self-awareness, and he started to see himself more clearly—without self-hatred or judgment. He found he was creative, kind, independent, thoughtful, an overall good person. During our sessions, I would guide him back to our therapeutic conversation from intellectual soliloquies about movies, which he was grateful for because he complained of doing this routinely in conversations, often losing his listener. As he struggled to touch his own emotions in sessions, we were able to use his interest in screenplays to showcase the importance of emotional intelligence, because that's what captures an audience in a movie. He slowly began to build his ability to sense and feel the emotions beneath his intellectualizations of life. I helped him slow down and maintain focus on himself. During our time together, he internalized the skills of slowing down and redirecting his mind and practiced these in session while on ketamine.

Here is a partial transcript of our integration session, which demonstrates three phases, reflection, building, and practicing. He had been journaling for two weeks since the final ketamine session. As the integration session began, I asked him for his reflections on what had healed and where his growth was. He said:

> I'm not so quick on the jump to feeling negative emotions, maybe a little more patient.

I have increased that buffer time to be intentional and aware, where I'm at, why I'm reacting this way. That has definitely helped.

Remember when I said "I'm different, but I'm okay" in the last session? I used to say it a lot, but it didn't really ring true until now. Since then it feels like it is even truer almost. This has helped me understand myself better, why I acted certain ways in the past.

I've been looking at neurodivergent coping skills, and that is helping.

Regarding productivity, I get into a slump, when I want to make something but can't, I get disheartened. It's good to know there are different ways of getting to an endpoint that work for me, ways that help me be more efficient. I had all the intentions, but it was never going to get to be efficient. Now I can put that intention into a different outlet.... I go into things with a different approach now, and that's been the whole issue for me. Having a more open mindset and be calm, approach things with more insight.

I have a better outlook on things. This thing isn't going exactly how I want it to be going, but I can now deal with it better, much easier for me not to get upset over the little things. Little things would have been just picked up and made me overwhelmed.

I feel less insecure, being more comfortable going out and doing things, and not worrying about how I am perceived at all times by all people. I'm more cognizant that everybody is doing their own thing, and nobody cares.

I am also getting along with my roommate, which was a one-way problem. I would get so annoyed over little things. But now I just don't think about that stuff much anymore. I am not hyper-focusing on it anymore.

I am also silencing and defeating the negative thoughts, but I'm still struggling with stating what I need and being more confident. I am not where I want to be.

Nature helps the most; reading helps cause it's quieter and less stimulated than movies and TVs that I am constantly looking at. I want to implement meditation into my day. And the same with yoga, but there are so many different ways to go about it. Learning not to get overwhelmed with all that, there's too much so I won't start kind of thing. I will just look at a few types and give it a try. I also want to write more, like journaling, or starting to work on my screenplays. I want a way to get my ideas down so I can stay focused and mindful of the present, so I don't get so lost in my head.

Moving forward, I think I would like to come for booster sessions, but I know it really depends on the work I put into myself more than the ketamine.

I am so proud of the work he put into his own growth. He came very prepared for his integration session. His therapy lasted roughly seven weeks, from the initial consultation through the final integration session, and now he is on his way to turning his attention from his distress toward living his aspirations. And as he stated, it's an ongoing practice, so I look forward to seeing his progress and supporting him during challenges.

As I close this chapter, I would like to share a personal example of the positive impacts of sustained practice, as humbling as this is. These experiences occurred while I was literally writing this chapter (of course they would!).

I was overjoyed to be in Portugal researching for and writing this book when a good friend called alerting me that an old adversary of mine, someone who caused great harm to my community and me some years back, had surfaced again after several quiet years, although

I had no idea what the person wanted. Immediately I felt alone and scared, like a child lost in the woods. I could feel myself shake, and my mind flooded with horrible scenarios, which just reinforced the fear. I was in trauma mode, and far from home.

In the past, this would have ruined my trip and sent me into hiding for some time. I saw all this happening and started to go into panic. My mind suggested using many of my old, unhealthy coping habits for fear and panic, but those would definitely ruin the trip. I kindly said to myself, *Didn't you just write about the power of practice? How would you move from trauma to triumph, Mikey?* I calmed myself with deep breathing, hands on heart and belly. I would not allow any person to control me or my experience or allow myself to be moved into panic by my own thoughts. Then I drew sweet and funny pictures of my dog and started laughing. Within ten minutes of experiencing emotions, thoughts, and constricting sensations that could have taken me down, I returned to joy with the help of my best friend, my imagination, and some creativity (all of which are in my ecosystem of change).

The inner ordeal passed, and I felt strong and grounded, an incredible benefit of this grounding and empowerment practice. I was again in command of my mind's attention, which I placed back on my experience of joy and wonder at being in Portugal. If fear rose again, I soothed myself and turned my attention back to living my life.

This is what dedicated practice gives us. Freedom—not from the pains of life but from the suffering of wallowing in them.

CHAPTER 11

EMBODIMENT
THE ART OF AUTHENTICITY

We have come to the end of our journey together, but you are just at the start of the rest of your life. We have come to a place where we can put our shoes in the closet, hang up our jacket, wash our worn and soiled clothing, eat a warm meal, and get a good night's sleep in our own bed. When we wake up, we will be home, where our soul feels safe and has room to breathe, to be creative and feel inspired. The pains of life will always come and go, but we now live in our heart space, and our suffering is so much less.

What is the point of this whole process if not to feel at home within ourselves and to live a life worth living?

Embodiment is the *feeling* of being at home, inside our own mind, body, and heart.

This chapter points toward what an embodied life can look and feel like. After all, we don't just want relief from symptoms. We want to flow in life with ease. To feel confident in who we are, and to live following our heart's values. To make wise choices and skillfully correct or repair when we don't. And to be fully authentic.

Embodiment is both the culmination of a process and the start of a new way of being. We are embodying what was always present, but not accessible. Of course, the process truly has no "culmination" but continues on and on and on. As with life, our process of transformation is fluid and continuous. This new way of being is ever unfolding. Even my most revered teachers in their mid-seventies have work to do. Being human is being messy. This is the way.

There is no stopping point for our growth, but things do get easier. The volume on our symptoms, old reactions, and miserable thoughts gets turned down as newer, healthier responses are created and integrated. "After" your integration phase, you become more attuned to your needs and meet them for yourself. This creates confidence, assuredness, and inner strength—all together being embodiment.

Each of us is capable of living deeply and embodying our highest potentials and values, all while feeling at home in ourselves. When the changes derived from the therapeutic process are more fully rooted and a new well-being baseline is set, we can move through the world empowered, at peace, and with more ease.

Living deeply is applied embodiment. It occurs when we think, act, and speak from a place that is deeply grounded in our own wise heart. This applies to all life circumstances: relationships, employment, community involvement, parenting, and so forth. When you are in a place of alignment with your heart and soul, and no longer live from or within any patchwork personas, you will operate and function in your life from a place of confidence and empowerment. This is embodying your values as well as living your life deeply. They go hand in hand.

Once you commit to and carry out the daily practices you chose during the integration phase, the changes you were seeking become a part of your identity and the new foundation for the self you are becoming. These changes are felt in the body, down to your cells.

In their book *Telomere Effect: A Revolutionary Approach to Living Younger, Healthier, Longer,* Nobel laureate Dr. Elizabeth Blackburn and stress psychologist Dr. Elissa Epel demonstrate that cells respond to changes in the environment and to our thoughts, beliefs, and behaviors. When we discover, speak, and live our truths, we literally *feel more alive* and embody a sense of deep calm while being less prone to sickness and disease. Living our truths is actually good for our health. Walking around the world feeling what we know about ourselves to be true is good medicine.

I am whole. I am kind. I am at peace. I believe in myself. I deserve to be heard and seen. I belong. Choose one truth you hold dear about yourself, and feel it in your body. Where do you feel it? Imagine walking into a room radiating that truth and authenticity—what would others feel? How would you feel walking into that room?

The changes we experience are felt physiologically, psychologically, energetically, and spiritually and are noticed and felt by others. We are different, more expanded, confident, wiser, kinder, and more understanding. When we are embodied, we naturally live more deeply and fully. Our lives become richer and more vibrant.

One male client in his fifties came to me feeling hopeless and depressed and with existential dread after the breakup of a nineteen-year relationship. He said that after his second ketamine session with me, his friends and family asked what had happened to him that he was so alive and happy! I noticed this, too, when I walked into the room before the third session. His eyes shone and seemed more alive. He attributed this change to the work we had done.

As a very young child, he'd become the caretaker of his other siblings and had to grow up quickly to survive. His feelings and needs were suppressed and ignored for the benefit of others, starting around six years of age. This was a habit he continued in his life, living in a persona of someone trained to think only of others. He was disconnected from himself, his dreams, his emotions, and even his own imagination. In two sessions, he not only realized this but also reconnected to himself after understanding why his partner said he was emotionally unavailable to her. He formed a new, healthy and loving relationship with himself, including his imagination and feelings, which left him feeling elated and excited. This is what his friends and family saw. It was beautiful to witness.

The idea is to *feel* life, not just think about it. And to feel, we need a body with its senses turned on and paid attention to. Living in our mind is exactly like eating a menu to taste the food. Life as an idea is dull. Have you ever seen videos of people who are deaf receiving implants and then they get to hear sounds for the first time in their life? It is so deeply moving to watch. To see their awe, astonishment, gratitude, and grief, all felt simultaneously, is magic and hurts a little too. This is often how my clients describe waking up to both their inner life and the grandeur of the universe. They become overwhelmed as their senses come online, their defenses dissolve, their hearts open, and they feel alive, sometimes for the first time in their life. They flood with grief, gratitude, hope, and relief. They *are* alive, after all!

It is hard to fully feel alive when we cut off our emotions to "protect" ourselves from feeling the uncomfortable or distressing ones. We feel alive when we actually sense those emotions, despite not liking them, while connecting with our body. To get to experience the positive emotions we are yearning for, we have to be open to all emotions. There is no way around this truth. Feeling is feeling. We don't get to pick and choose what we feel if we want to feel. Embodiment is being full of life.

In psychedelic psychotherapy, we welcome and accept the feelings we have avoided. There is a healthy immersion into the depths of our feelings while we also maintain the stance of being a witness. This is very much like mindfulness practice, when we experience what arises in the moment while bearing witness to it. This also aligns with the nondual practice of being both this and that, experiencer and witness of the experience. This is why I consider psychedelic psychotherapy to be a spiritual practice as well as a therapy. We learn to welcome and tolerate distressing emotions with equanimity while developing the capacity to be still and mindful no matter what arises within us. This is necessary for an embodied life.

If we want to feel joy, we also need to feel sadness.

Bliss? Then anguish.

Happiness? Grief then.

All of it comes with all of it. And it's actually better this way.

In my work, distressing emotions bring valuable information that something is misaligned in a client's life, and so in psychedelic psychotherapy we learn to greet and honor them as they arise in session. And from these experiences in session, new skills are built. Embodiment is carrying what you need to handle life's challenges within you: emotional tolerance, acceptance of life just as it is, wisdom, insight, clarity, truth, honesty, authenticity, patience, and compassion, just to name a few. And these are discovered during the active process of healing while engaged in psychedelic psychotherapy and put to use afterward.

The therapeutic journey through the entire process is not just healing but also training. Much like when Luke met with Yoda to prepare himself to fulfill his destiny, psychedelic psychotherapy is really like Jedi training with healing embedded in it. You are better able to face life's challenges and build resiliency, confidence, trust in yourself, and strength, without being brought down by troubles. All this was in you the whole time, you just had to find it and bring it to the surface during your healing journey.

Please indulge me one more *Star Wars* mention. If you watch Luke closely during the original three movies, you will see his transformation—from a snot-nosed, whiny farm boy to an embodied spiritual warrior. At first, his strength was limited, because it was based on his own muscle and ego, which could not match his life circumstances. It was through his commitment to inner psychospiritual training and his deep connection to the mysterious forces of the universe that he transformed. (I do have to say, though, Princess Leia was empowered and embodied from the start, so maybe we should be following her lead instead? Just saying.)

EMBODIMENT PRACTICE

Here are some qualities of an embodied person: attentive, present, compassionate, mindful, flexible, adaptable, kind with firm boundaries, gentle yet a fierce advocate when they need to be, someone with a presence, with integrity, and with the ability to laugh at themselves. They radiate. Can you think of any embodied people in your life? Someone who inspires you to be the best version of yourself? Someone who exudes presence when near them?

Take a moment and think of them, and sense your body's response. When do you show up this way? Would you come to mind as the embodied person for anyone in your life? Would you like to? I believe psychedelic psychotherapy not only helps us heal but also can transform us into people who have a positive impact on others just through presence.

EMBODYING OUR ETHICS

Many years ago, my ex-wife and I used to lead dharma and cultural trips to Thailand, where I did my Peace Corps service and where she grew up. One year we invited my teacher, Richard Miller, to join us to lead the spiritual practices during the trip. On one morning, we brought all our guests and Richard to a Buddhist temple to meet with the head monk, who was a renowned dharma teacher in the region. After a meditation practice, I led a discussion between the two teachers to demonstrate the differences and similarities of two distinct world spiritual traditions. My last question to both of these incredible, embodied teachers was "What is the ultimate goal of your practice?"

I was expecting answers about enlightenment and serene spiritual states. What they said humbled and surprised me. Richard said, "Be kind, be kind, be kind," and laughed. Ajahn M. said, "Do good, and try not to cause harm," and also laughed.

This moment changed my perception of what it means to be "spiritual." One who embodies their ethics and values is enlightened. It has taken me many years of practice since then, while humbly cleaning up a lot of mistakes I've made, to understand this teaching. It was a very powerful reminder that a life lived deeply is one based on turning virtue and ethics into actions.

When my clients really start to see themselves more clearly, they begin to lose their attachment to behaviors that are harmful to themselves and others. They just don't tolerate things that no longer serve them or that are detrimental to their own and others' health. To paraphrase Jack Kornfield, it's hard to maintain a spiritual life when you're still lying to yourself.

I'm sure you've heard of the Tao Te Ching, a collection of teachings by the Chinese sage Lao Tzu. The *Te* is made up of two characters: virtue (upright heart) and stepping out (left foot), which together mean "virtue in action." The basis of Taoism is bringing harmony and balance to one's inner life, which is then expressed outwardly through skillful and compassionate actions. This mirrors the term *praxis* that Paulo Freire coined in his seminal text *Pedagogy of the Oppressed*. He means the application of theory to an action, because both are necessary when working toward purposeful and meaningful social change. Ideas and concepts about social or environmental change without action is the same as having personal insights without the necessary behavior changes. Nothing changes or gets done. For purposeful change to occur within ourselves, in our society, and on the planet, we have to apply what we've learned. How else are humanity's troubles going to be transformed?

One of the most powerful changes I've seen in psychedelic psychotherapy occurred with a police officer. All the first responders I work with care tremendously about and are dedicated to serving their community. These men and women who, day after day, year in and year out, don their uniforms to rescue, help, support, keep safe, heal, and protect the public in the face of grave and life-threatening danger do so out of their deep inner commitment to service. Their uniforms are an external symbol of their unwavering dedication, strength, and resiliency in light of the reoccurring traumas they face in the line of duty.

In many cases, first responders are great examples of what embodying ethics looks like. (Of course, I am greatly aware of the serious and life-threatening misuse of power and force that some police officers have engaged in to the harm of African Americans specifically. Reform and implicit bias training are desperately warranted. And it is important to acknowledge that the great majority of officers spend their shifts going on calls to protect women and children in domestic violence situations, to work with the chronically ill homeless population, and to mitigate situations that most of us could not stomach or handle, on our behalf. With power comes great responsibility, and there is much room for growth.)

The police officer I worked with realized his resolve to protect his community from violence and serious harm was fused with the anger he felt toward the perpetrators. He was a fierce protector of women and children and would often feel anger for days after a call in which he had to rescue someone from the terrible grip of violence. His blood pressure and heart rate would stay elevated long after his calls, and a sound sleep was nearly impossible.

In his healing journey, compassion for his own traumas and wounds grew. His compassion for and understanding of others also blossomed. He started to see himself in others, and others in him. He saw how his anger was reasonable but not necessary to do his job well. Using force without anger became a possibility.

This subtle but immensely significant shift moved him from someone who could potentially abuse his power "in the service of protecting" to one who more fully embodied his highest ethics.

Ethics is the foundation of a good life.

For all of us.

Psychedelic psychotherapy gives us an opportunity to very clearly see ourselves, our behaviors, and our harmful beliefs. This process allows us to better understand our impact on ourselves and others, to atone, and to repair where appropriate.

If all that psychedelic psychotherapy did is create more embodied, ethical people, then our world would dramatically shift toward more peace. As a Zen monk, I occasionally wear my full robes, which are a symbol of my dedication to peace, love, understanding, awakening, and service. This is the uniform I don to remind myself to stay in integrity and embody the ethics I vowed to keep.

You don't have to be a Buddhist monk or a first responder to aspire to embody your ethics. What I found is most of my clients who go through psychedelic psychotherapy naturally become more aware of their ethics, behavior, and impact. After all, most of them were deeply wounded, traumatized, and hurt by others *not* embodying theirs. It is clear that once a client truly heals these old wounds, they become advocates and allies of others and, most importantly, of themselves.

COLLECTIVE EMBODIMENT

The issues we face as a species, the ones we've created out of greed, hatred, and ignorance, can only shift when we collectively awaken to our shared responsibility for all life on this planet. We all have the potential to be effective, emboldened, empowered, and embodied humans. Even if the extent of one's contribution and impact is within a small family, that can be enough to train the next generation to be mindful and conscious of the preciousness and fragility of life. My clients who are parents tell me how much the PP process has given them new perspectives not only on how to parent but also on what to teach their children about their relationship to the larger world. As more parents, who are themselves healing and transforming, embody the principles they teach to their children, the future will begin to shift toward those ethics. This is one way psychedelic psychotherapy is starting to make an impact on collective transformation and well-being.

Collective transformation happens through us, as together we create the outer reality found deep within our wise and loving hearts. Psychedelic psychotherapy may be one key to resolving many of the problems we face around the world because it unlocks our innate wisdom and compassion that we then turn into skillful actions. Imagine when embodied people start to take the lead in our political systems. We want those who live deeply and who are committed to virtue and ethics making the vital decisions on behalf of our communities and the planet. In doing this personal work, we will lead by living fully and being authentic. From this place, we can influence the collective consciousness of all humanity toward the harmony and balance we so long for.

Let's send our world leaders, politicians, lawmakers, religious leaders, prison wardens, police chiefs, high-ranking military officers, and CEOs to psychedelic psychotherapy. In fact, that should be a prerequisite before they are sworn in, take office, or are allowed to hold so much power and influence.

I will even clear my schedule for them. ☺

Let's get ourselves healthy, embodied, empowered, and authentic. First, this is our natural state. Second, the world needs us to be who we were meant to be.

Remember, you don't have to take a psychedelic to discover, speak, and live your truth. You can start right now. Ask your heart what it truly longs for, and don't deny what you hear. Just listen and consider it:

Listen with your full attention.
Listen like an angel or God or an ancestor is speaking to you.
Listen like your future depends on it, because it does.

Learning to listen to your own soul is like sitting in a forest and hearing the diverse sounds of life—the cawing of a raven, the chitter of a squirrel, wind through leaves, pine cones dropping to earth, the babbling of a nearby stream. Your soul has a sacred sound that rings like a bell when its truth is spoken.

This secret is yours to learn if you slow down, bring your attention inward, refrain from judging what you hear, and welcome what you see.

Own it, it is you, after all, who is yearning for your own attention. All parts of you are needed to live a fully embodied life of authenticity, which is the key to good mental health.

The medicine and psychotherapeutic support accelerate this process, but all this is already inside you. Waiting to be discovered and brought forward.

It's up to you.

I hope this book and the teachings within have helped you on your path to knowing how precious this life is, how important you are, and how you have within you what you need to live deeply. You are good, whole, and unbroken. Your essence is pure and innocent. And the world is waiting on you to fully step into the person you were born to be.

You are worthy of unconditional love, right in this very moment, for no reason at all.

Now go live!
Thank you for reading.

YOU ARE ENOUGH.

YOU ALWAYS HAVE BEEN.

Falling Upward into Grace

*We usually think of the Fall
as moving downward
rapidly through space
upside down,
arms flailing,
hands grasping,
mouth agape,
in a soundless
scream.*

But whose dream is this anyway?

*I'd prefer falling upward into Grace.
Like when a baby is tossed
high into the air
as if she were a beach ball
delighted to be lifted
into the heavens,
past birds,
through clouds,
finally reaching
the vast dark
of space.*

*Quiet,
peaceful,
infinite.*

QUESTIONS TO ASK A PSYCHEDELIC PSYCHOTHERAPIST WHEN YOU ARE CONSIDERING TREATMENT

When you are ready to seek out psychedelic-assisted therapy, you'll want to research the therapist and have a discussion with them about their orientation, protocols, and safety measures. Here is a short list of questions you can use as a guide to assessing potential therapists:

- What is your background in psychedelic psychotherapy? How long have you been practicing? With whom did you train and for how long?
- What do you focus on in your work? Do you have experience working with . . . ?
- How does spirituality play a role in this work, and do you come from any specific tradition?
- What can I expect from this therapy?
- What does the preparation phase look like?
- What does your integration plan or process look like?
- What ethical guidelines do you use or follow in your work?
- What safety measures do you have in place? How do you handle any medical or psychiatric issues or emergencies?
- What is your policy on touch and sexuality?

RESOURCES

Blackburn, Elizabeth H., and Elissa Epel. *The Telomere Effect: A Revolutionary Approach to Living Younger, Healthier, Longer.* Orion Spring, 2018.
Chadwick, David. *To Shine One Corner of the World: Moments with Shunryu Suzuki.* Broadway Books, 2001.
Chödrön, Pema. *Welcoming the Unwelcome: Wholehearted Living in a Brokenhearted World.* Shambhala, 2020.
Epel, Elissa. *The Telomere Effect.* Grand Central Publishing, 2017.
Fadiman, James. *The Psychedelic Explorer's Guide: Safe, Therapeutic, and Sacred Journeys.* Park Street Press, 2011.
Grof, Stanislav, and Christina Grof. *Spiritual Emergency: When Personal Transformation Becomes a Crisis.* Tarcher, 1989.
Hart, Carl L. *Drug Use for Grown-Ups: Chasing Liberty in the Land of Fear.* Penguin Books, 2022.
Haupt, Lyanda Lynn, and Helen Nicholson. *Rooted: Life at the Crossroads of Science, Nature, and Spirit.* Little, Brown Spark, 2023.
Hayes, Steven. *Get Out of Your Mind and into Your Life: The New Acceptance and Commitment Therapy.* New Harbinger Publications, 2022.
Holger, Kalweit. *Shamans, Healers and Medicine Men.* Shambhala, 2001.
Jung, C. G., and R. F. C. Hull. *The Undiscovered Self: The Dilemma of the Individual in Modern Society.* Signet, 2006.
Kimmerer, Robin Wall. *Braiding Sweetgrass: Indigenous Wisdom, Scientific Knowledge, and the Teachings of Plants.* Milkweed Editions, 2015.
Kornfield, Jack. *After the Ecstasy, the Laundry: How the Heart Grows Wise on the Spiritual Path.* Bantam Books, 2001.
Kornfield, Jack. *Still Forest Pool.* 1997.
Kornfield, Jack, and Paul Breiter. *Still Forest Pool: The Insight Meditation of Achaan Chah.* Quest Books, 2013.
Lamb, F. Bruce, and Andrew Weil. *Wizard of the Upper Amazon: The Story of Manuel Córdova-Rios.* North Atlantic Books, 1986.
Luke, David, and Rory Spowers. *DMT Entity Encounters: Dialogues on the Spirit Molecule with Ralph Metzner, Chris Bache, Jeffrey Kripal, Whitley Strieber, Angela Voss, and Others.* Park Street Press, 2021.

Metzner, Ralph. *The Unfolding Self: Varieties of Transformative Experience.* Synergetic Press, 2022.

Michael, Coby. *The Poison Path Herbal: Baneful Herbs, Medicinal Nightshades, and Ritual Entheogens.* Park Street Press, 2021.

Miller, Madeline. *Circe.* Bloomsbury, 2023.

Pendell, Dale. *Pharmako Gnosis: Plant Teachers and the Poison Path.* North Atlantic Books, 2010.

Pollan, Michael. *How to Change Your Mind: What the New Science of Psychedelics Teaches Us About Consciousness, Dying, Addiction, Depression, and Transcendence.* Penguin Books, 2019.

Prechtel, Martín. *The Smell of Rain on Dust: Grief and Praise.* North Atlantic Books, 2015.

Read, Tim, and Jules Evans. *Breaking Open: Finding a Way Through Spiritual Emergencies.* Aeon Books, 2020.

Read, Tim, and Maria Papaspyrou. *Psychedelics and Psychotherapy: The Healing Potential of Expanded States.* Park Street Press, 2021.

Richards, William A. *Sacred Knowledge: Psychedelics and Religious Experiences.* Columbia University Press, 2016.

Roszak, Theodore, Mary E. Gomes, and Allen D. Kanner, eds. *Ecopsychology: Restoring the Earth, Healing the Mind.* Sierra Club Books, 1995.

Schwartz, Richard C. *No Bad Parts: How the Internal Family Systems Model Changes Everything.* Sounds True, 2021.

Smith, Huston. *Cleansing the Doors of Perception: The Religious Significance of Entheogenic Plants and Chemicals.* Sentient Publications, 2003.

Starr, Mirabai. *Ordinary Mysticism: Your Life as Sacred Ground.* Harper One, 2024.

Strassman, Rick. *DMT: The Spirit Molecule.* Park Street Press, 2001.

Swan, Laura. *The Forgotten Desert Mothers: Sayings, Lives, and Stories of Early Christian Women.* Paulist Press, 2022.

Tarnas, Richard. *Cosmos and Psyche: Intimations of a New World View.* Plume, 2007.

Walsh, Roger. *World of Shamanism: New Views of an Ancient Tradition.* BookBaby, 2024.

Weller, Francis. *The Wild Edge of Sorrow: Rituals of Renewal and the Sacred Work of Grief.* North Atlantic Books, 2021.

NOTES

Introduction to Psychedelic Psychotherapy

1. Please check out an amazing short film I am in called *An Act of Service*. It is directed by Brandon Kapelow and features Captain Rob Christensen of the Boise Fire Department.

2. "MDMA-Assisted Therapy for PTSD: Open-Label Lead-In Study (MP16)," Multidisciplinary Association for Psychedelic Studies, https://maps.org/mdma/ptsd/lead-in; "MDMA-Assisted Therapy for PTSD: Boulder, Colorado (MP12)," Multidisciplinary Association for Psychedelic Studies, https://maps.org/mdma/ptsd/boulder; Jennifer Dore, Brent Turnipseed, Shannon Dwyer, Andrea Turnipseed, Julane Andries, German Ascani, et al., "Ketamine Assisted Psychotherapy (KAP): Patient Demographics, Clinical Data and Outcomes in Three Large Practices Administering Ketamine with Psychotherapy," *Journal of Psychoactive Drugs* 51, no. 2 (2019): 189–198, https://pubmed.ncbi.nlm.nih.gov/30917760; and Sandra J. Drozdz, Akash Goel, Matthew W. McGarr, Joel Katz, Paul Ritvo, Gabriella F Mattina, et al., "Ketamine Assisted Psychotherapy: A Systematic Narrative Review of the Literature," *Journal of Pain Research* 15 (2022): 1691–1706, https://pubmed.ncbi.nlm.nih.gov/35734507.

3. Yes, there are truly debilitating mental health disorders that make even the simplest daily activities challenging for some. For those folks, really good psychosocial treatments and important medications are available to consider to help stabilize.

4. Entheogens are psychoactive substances used in sacred contexts to induce spiritual development.

5. A note on the difference between *legalization* and *decriminalization*. Legalization occurs when state governments or the federal government passes laws and legislation making once-banned or illegal drugs legal for use. With decriminalization, the use of a drug is still prohibited, but the legal system will not punish for possession of up to a certain amount of that drug. Although decriminalization is an important step in the process, it does not allow the drug to be used therapeutically or legally.

Chapter 2: Medicine and the Power of Truth

1. Shawn Ziff, Benjamin Stern, Gregory Lewis, Maliha Majeed, and Vasavi Rakesh Gorantla, "Analysis of Psilocybin-Assisted Therapy in Medicine: A Narrative Review," *Cureus* 14, no. 2 (2022): e21944, https://doi.org/10.7759/cureus.21944.

2. Ziff et al., "Analysis of Psilocybin-Assisted Therapy in Medicine," e21944.

3. Ziff et al., "Analysis of Psilocybin-Assisted Therapy in Medicine," e21944; and Leslie Morland and Joshua Woolley, "PTSD: National Center for PTSD: Psychedelic-Assisted Therapy for PTSD," Department of Veterans Affairs, March 28, 2024, www.ptsd.va.gov/professional/treat/txessentials/psychedelics_assisted_therapy.asp#three.

4. "5-MeO-DMT Therapy Information—UC Berkeley BCSP," UC Berkeley Center for the Science of Psychedelics, May 17, 2023, psychedelics.berkeley.edu/substance/5-meo-dmt; Robert B. Kargbo, "5-MeO-DMT: Potential Use of Psychedelic-Induced Experiences in the Treatment of Psychological Disorders," *ACS Medicinal Chemistry Letters* 12, no. 11 (2021): 1646–1648, https://doi.org/10.1021/acsmedchemlett.1c00546; and Anna O. Ermakova, Fiona Dunbar, James Rucker, and Matthew W. Johnson, "A Narrative Synthesis of Research with 5-MeO-DMT," *Journal of Psychopharmacology* 36, no. 3 (2021): 273–294, https://doi.org/10.1177/02698811211050543.

5. Juan José Fuentes, Francina Fonesca, Matilde Elices, Magí Farré, and Marta Torrens, "Therapeutic Use of LSD in Psychiatry: A Systematic Review of Randomized-Controlled Clinical Trials," *Frontiers in Psychiatry* 10 (2020), https://doi.org/10.3389/fpsyt.2019.00943; and Bryce D. Beutler, Kenneth Shinozuka, Burton J. Tabaac, Alejandro Arenas, Kirsten Cherian, and Viviana D. Evans, et al., "Psychedelic Therapy: A Primer for Primary Care Clinicians—Lysergic Acid Diethylamide (LSD)," *American Journal of Therapeutics* 31, no. 2 (2024): e104–e111, https://doi.org/10.1097/MJT.0000000000001726.

6. Stephen J. Hyde, *Ketamine for Depression* (Xlibris, 2015); Steven B. Rosenbaum, Vikas Gupta, Preeti Patel, and Jorge L. Palacios, *Ketamine* (StatPearls Publishing, 2024), www.ncbi.nlm.nih.gov/books/NBK470357; and H. Valerie Curran and Lisa Monaghan, "In and Out of the K-Hole: A Comparison of the Acute and Residual Effects of Ketamine in Frequent and Infrequent Ketamine Users," *Addiction* 96, no. 5 (2001): 749–760, https://doi.org/10.1046/j.1360-0443.2001.96574910.x.

7. Daniel F. Jiménez-Garrido, María Gómez-Sousa, Genís Ona, Rafael G. Dos Santos, Jaime E. C. Hallak, Miguel Ángel Alcázar-Córcoles, et al., "Effects of Ayahuasca on Mental Health and Quality of Life in Naïve Users: A Longitudinal and Cross-Sectional Study Combination," *Scientific Reports* 10, art. 4075 (2020), https://doi.org/10.1038/s41598-020-61169-x; and Ede Frecska, Petra

Bokor, and Michael Winkelman, "The Therapeutic Potentials of Ayahuasca: Possible Effects Against Various Diseases of Civilization," *Frontiers in Pharmacology* 7 (2016), https://doi.org/10.3389/fphar.2016.00035.

8. "Traditional Medicine Has a Long History of Contributing to Conventional Medicine and Continues to Hold Promise," World Health Organization, August 10, 2023, www.who.int/news-room/feature-stories/detail/traditional-medicine-has-a-long-history-of-contributing-to-conventional-medicine-and-continues-to-hold-promise.

Chapter 8: Psyche and Cosmos

1. Carl G. Jung and R. F. C. Hull, *The Undiscovered Self: The Dilemma of the Individual in Modern Society* (Signet, 2006), 101.

2. A. Marks, L. J. Brazier, D. Singer, M. Kirch, E. Solway, S. Roberts, E. Smith, L. Hutchens, P. Malani, and J. Kullgren, "Religious and Spiritual Beliefs and Health Care," University of Michigan National Poll on Healthy Aging, December 2022, https://dx.doi.org/10.7302/6642.

INDEX

Acceptance and Commitment Therapy (ACT), 203–204
achievement, COVID pandemic and shifting focus to authenticity from, 86–88
aftercare, 131–132
After the Ecstasy, the Laundry (Kornfield), 200
agency, retention of during psychedelic psychotherapy, 80, 120
alignment, 74–86
  authenticity and, 74, 86–89
  consciously choosing and, 78
  with core values, 77–78
  with our body, 83–86
  with our future, 79–82
  with our intuition and wisdom, 78–79
  with true identity and innocence, 75–77
ancestral domain
  preparation sessions and, 101, 104–106
  role in psychedelic psychotherapy, 13–15
ancestry, ceremonial uses of psychedelics and, 38–39
Antonini, Clair, 107
anxiety, 5, 9
  psychedelic treatment for, 12, 13, 16, 29, 30, 33, 36
applied mysticism, 185–188
archetypes, 163–164, 169–170, 171–173, 175
  defined, 169
Arjuna and Krishna, story of, 148
art therapy, 134
attention, practice and, 205, 206, 208
authenticity, 11

alignment and, 74, 86–89
  COVID pandemic and shift in focus from achievement to, 86–88
  See also embodiment
ayahuasca, 35–37
ayahuasca retreats, 38
ayahuasca vine (*Banisteriopsis caapi*), 35
Ayurveda medicine, 141

"bad trip," 26, 154–155
bearing witness as therapeutic response, 159–161
Becker, Gavin de, 84
beliefs
  about self, conditioned, 4–5, 42–43, 52–53, 55, 59, 72–74, 78, 102–103, 142–143, 159
  spiritual, 103–104, 147, 149–150, 157
belonging, psychedelic psychotherapy and increasing sense of, 4, 5, 12, 24, 103–104, 164, 174, 185, 190
Bhagavad Gita, 148
Blackburn, Elizabeth, 216–217
body
  aligning with your, 83–86
  feeling change, 216–220
  preparing to enter the temple and, 117
"body keeps the score," 83
brain, effect of psychedelic medicines on, 6, 7, 10, 148–149
Breaking Open (Evans), 200
Buddhist psychology, 19
Bufo alvarius (Colorado River or Sonoran Desert toad), 27, 28

INDEX

Cahn, Rael, 8–9
calm, returning to place of during psychedelic sessions, 149
Carhart-Harris, Robin, 8–9
ceremonial uses of psychedelics, 38–40
chacruna shrub (*Psychotria viridis*), 35
Chah, Ajahn, 116
challenging experiences during psychedelic sessions, 136–161
   "bad trips," 26, 154–155
   conditions calling for therapeutic attention during, 13
   interpersonal, 152–154
   physiological and somatic, 140–142
   psychological, 142–147
   safety, 155–159
   spirituality, 147–152
   vomiting, 138–139
change
   embodying ethics and, 220–223
   feeling, 217–220
   psychedelic psychotherapy facilitating, 16–17
Chodron, Pema, 139
Circe (Miller), 169–170
clients
   relationship with therapist, 98–99, 152–154, 159–161
   safety during sessions and, 155–159
collective embodiment, 223–225
coming down from psychedelic session, 130–131
community, practice and, 205, 207, 209
conditioning and programming, reflecting on original face beneath, 73–74, 75. *See also* alignment; beliefs
connection, psychedelic psychotherapy and feeling, 5, 24, 48, 141, 164–165, 174. *See also* belonging
core values, aligning with, 77–78
cosmos
   consciousness of, 173–176
   encountering and embracing in session, 176–178

COST stance, 111–114, 123
   curiosity, 111–112
   openness, 112
   surrender, 112–113
   trust, 114
countertransference, 153
COVID pandemic, changes in careers and relationships and, 86–88
cultural genogram, 104
curanderos/curanderas, 39
curating lifestyle activities in integration phase, 200–201, 203–209
curiosity, COST stance and, 111–112

death, relationship with, 104, 188–191
deep breathing, 104
default mode network (DMN), psychedelic medicines and, 6, 7, 10, 148–149
depression, 5, 9
   psychedelic treatment for, 12, 13, 25, 27, 30, 32–33, 35
depth therapy, 4
dharma gates, psychedelic psychotherapy and, 11–12, 128
dharma trips, 220–221
dimethyltryptamine (DMT), 35
domains of psychedelic psychotherapy, 5–6, 101–106
   ancestral, 13–15, 101, 104–106
   See also physiological domain; psychological domain; spiritual domain
dopamine, ketamine and, 7, 33
dosing psychedelics
   ayahuasca, 36
   determining dose, 44–46
   5-MeO-DMT, 27
   ketamine, 33–34
   LSD, 31
   MDMA, 29
   psilocybin, 25
   safety during sessions and, 156
Dune (Herbert), 195

Ecosystem of Change, 203, 204–205
ecosystem of support, building,
    202–205
"ego death," 118
ego dissolution, 118, 129–130
    bad reactions to, 139
    bad trips and, 154–155
    helping client deal with, 148–150
    innate healing intelligence and, 115
    psychedelic psychotherapy and, 4,
        5, 10–15
embodiment, 215–225
    collective, 223–225
    defined, 215
    embodying our ethics, 220–223
    feeling change, 216–220
    of lifestyle changes, 205–209
    living deeply as applied, 216
    qualities of embodied person, 220
empathogen, MDMA as, 28–29
empowerment
    informed consent process and, 98
    psychedelic therapy and, 120
entactogen, MDMA as, 28–29
Epel, Elissa, 217
epigenetics, ancestors/ancestral domain
    and, 13–14, 104
ethics, embodying our, 220–223
Ethics of Caring, The (Taylor), 99
Evans, Jules, 200
"everything all at once," 41, 176–178
exercises
    four domains, 105
    meditation and reflection on future
        self, 82–83
    patchwork persona personal
        reflection, 58–59
    on surrendering, 113
expectations about psychedelic
    psychotherapy, 110–111
experience given by psychedelic
    medicines, 23–24
exploratory questions, during psychedelic
    session, 124–125

"face of God," 176–178
fear
    curiosity countering, 111
    psychedelic psychotherapy and facing,
        11–12, 195–197
feeling change, 217–220
fire ceremony, 133
5-MeO-DMT, 27–28
    surrender and, 112–113
    use at retreat, 134, 180, 181
flashbacks, LSD, 31
Food and Drug Administration (FDA), 27, 30
Freire, Paulo, 221
futuremaking, 81
future self
    aligning with, 79–82
    finding through psychedelic
        psychotherapy, 72–74
    meditating and reflecting on, 82–83
    visualizing, 72–73
    See also alignment

Garcia-Fons, Renaud, 107
Gift of Fear, The (Becker), 84
goodness, path to discovering your
    innate, 73–74
grief, confronting during psychedelic
    session, 143–144
Grof, Stan and Christina, 200
group ceremonies, 39–40
guidance, practice and, 205, 206–207, 209

Haynes, Richard, 209
healing
    ancestral, 14–15
    innate healing intelligence, 114–116
    inner healer, 114–116
    nondual, 18–20
    during preparation sessions, 119–120
    psychedelic psychotherapy and, 21–22
    speaking one's truth and, 121–122
    spirituality and, 147–148
    subjective experience of person taking
        psychedelic and, 8–9

INDEX

"Heart Is the Hero" (Wood Brothers), 181
Herbert, Frank, 195
Hofmann, Albert, 32
Holocaust, epigenetic changes passed down from survivors of, 3
Hoshino, Toshio, 28
humility, curiosity and practicing, 112

identity
 aligning with true, 75–77
 losing in psychedelic session, 129–130
images
 cosmic, 176–178
 role in healing and transformation, 164, 167–169, 170
indigeneity, 38
indigenous, 38
informed consent process, 95, 97–99
 revealing therapists are mandated reporters, 147
inherited trauma, 104
innate healing intelligence, 114–116
inner child, innocence of, 68–69
inner-directed therapist, 40
inner-directed uses of psychedelics, 40–41
inner healer, 114–116
"inner resource," 149
inner voice, aligning with, 78–79
innocence, aligning with, 75–77
integration phase of psychedelic psychotherapy, 15, 195–214
 difficulties faced in, 199–200
 ecosystem of support and clarifying values, 199, 202–205
 example of, 210–214
 following retreat, 135
 integration plan, 200–209
 practicing what matters, 205–209
 realistic expectations for, 209–210
 reflection phase, 201–202
 reinforcing change, 197–199
intentions
 practice and, 205, 206, 208
 setting, 99–101, 111

interdependence and connection,
 psychedelic psychotherapy and feeling, 5, 24, 48, 141, 164–165, 174. *See also* belonging
intergenerational trauma, 104
Internal Family Systems (IFS) model, 15
intuition, alignment and, 78–79

journal/journaling
 preparing for psychedelic session, 105–106, 117
 reflecting after psychedelic session, 123, 131, 170, 201
journey notes, 122–123
joy, rediscovering, 106–109
Jung, Carl, 166

Kabat-Zin, Jon, 185
kanjis, 49–50
karma, 14
ketamine, 32–35
 determining dose, 44–45
 neuroscience of, 6–8
 physiological effects of, 6–7
 recreational use of, 34, 37–38
ketamine-assisted psychotherapy (KAP), 32–33, 97
ketamine clinic process, 96–97
Kornfield, Jack, 200, 221
Krishna and Arjuna, 148

Lao Tzu, 221
lifestyle activities, integration phase and, 200–209
Living Deeply (Schlitz, Vieten & Amorak), 205–206
love, psychedelic psychotherapy and applying to self, 12, 18, 70–74, 208–209
LSD (lysergic acid diethylamide), 8, 30–32

MDMA (methylenedioxymethamphetamine), 28–30
"medicine does what the medicine will," 103, 116

INDEX

medicine men/women, 39
meditation, 4, 104
  on future self, 82–83
  neuroscience of, 6
  nondual, 20
  preparing to enter the temple and, 117
  trust-building and surrender-oriented, 118
mental health, incorporating body into treating, 85. *See also* anxiety; depression
metaphors
  role in healing and transformation, 164
  subconscious speaking in, 128–129
Miller, Madeline, 169–170
Miller, Richard, 149, 220–221
mind, relinquishing control of working, 109
mind-body interdependence, 141–142
mindfulness, 19
  preparing for session and, 117, 123
misaligned life. *See* patchwork persona
misalignment
  negative self-beliefs creating, 4–5
  suffering and, 74
monoamine oxidase inhibitors (MAOIs), 35
mortality, facing, 188–191
Murray, William Hutchinson, 79–80
Museum of Us (San Diego), 46–47
mushrooms. *See* psilocybin
mysticism, 179–191
  applied, 185–188
  ordinary, 183, 185, 188–191

nature, feeling connection to, 168, 175
neuroscience of psychedelic psychotherapy, 6–9
"Nove alla Turca" (Garcia-Fons & Antonini), 107

"October" (Rasmusson), 108
openness, COST stance and, 112
ordinary mysticism, 183, 185, 188–191
original face, discovering your, 73–74, 75

patchwork persona
  default personas, 64–66
  examining in psychedelic psychotherapy, 55
  excavating the, 59–64
  formation of, 52–58
  innocence of inner child, 68–69
  journeying toward self-love, 70–74
  personal reflection exercise, 58–59
  truth as medicine and, 66–68
Pedagogy of the Oppressed (Freire), 221
personality formed in relation to others' beliefs, judgments, and opinions, 52–58
personal truths, 48–50
physiological domain
  challenging experiences during psychedelic sessions and, 137, 140–142
  preparation sessions and, 101, 102
  vomiting, 137–138
physiological effect of ketamine, 6–7
play, embodying a lost art of, 171–173
Postsecrets art project, 46–47, 145
practice, 205–209
  defined, 205–206
  depth of effect on the body, 216–217
  realistic expectations for, 209–210
praxis, 221
preparation, 93–120
  COST stance, 111–114
  dealing with expectations, 110–111
  four domains, 101–106
  healing possibilities in, 119–120
  informed consent and therapeutic relationship, 97–99
  initial prep sessions, 96–97
  inner healer and innate healing intelligence, 114–116
  intention setting, 99–101
  preparing to enter the temple, 116–117
  rediscovering joy, 106–109
  stepping inside the temple, 118–119

present moment
  moving toward being in the, 72
  power of, 184–185, 187–188
programming and conditioning, revealed
    during psychedelic psychotherapy, 50,
    66, 68, 72–74, 78, 126–127
projections between client and
    therapist, 153
prompts
  on aligning with one's future, 81–82
  reflection, 201–202
  to use with client faced with unwelcomed
    presence, 151
psilocybin, 8, 24–27
  determining dose, 45–46
  use at veterans' retreat, 133–134,
    180, 181
psyche, 162–178
  archetypes, 163–164, 169–173, 175
  cosmos, 173–178
  embodying art of play and sexuality,
    171–173
  face of god (everything all at once), 41,
    176–178
  shadow parts, 165
  symbols and raven lead the way, 167–169
  whole self, 166–167
psychedelic, defined, 46
psychedelic medicines
  ayahuasca, 35–37
  default mode network and, 6, 7, 10,
    148–149
  defined, 46
  defining truth and, 48–50
  dissolving and displacing ego and, 10–15
  LSD, 8, 30–32
  MDMA, 28–30
  power of truth and, 46–48
  proper relationship with, 23–24, 43–44
  uses of, 37–43
  See also dosing psychedelics;
    5-Meo-DMT; ketamine; psilocybin
psychedelic psychotherapy (PP), 41–43
  changes following, 16–17

determining dose, 44–46
discovering your innate goodness
    during, 73–74
facing fears, 11–12, 195–197
fourfold aim of, 12
healing voyage of, 21–22
neuroscience of, 6–9
nondual healing and, 18–20
offering direct experience of belonging
    and interconnectedness, 5, 164–165
psychotherapeutic, 41–43
retention of agency during, 80, 120
as somatically oriented therapy, 141–142
speaking one's truth and, 66–68,
    121–122
traditional therapy *vs.*, 4
well-being and, 4
working with "everything, everywhere, all
    at once," 41, 176–178
See also integration; transformation
psychedelic psychotherapy (PP) process,
    121–135
  aftercare, 131–132
  coming down, 130–131
  day of, 123–129
  ego dissolution, 129–130
  intro and grounding, 123
  journey notes, 122–123
  onset, 124
  prolonged effects of, 199–200
  retreats, 132–135
  signs, symbols, and metaphors, 128–129
  somatic awareness during a session, 128
  therapeutic exploration phase, 124–128
  truth arising during, 121–122
  wrap-up, 131–132
  See also challenging experiences during
    psychedelic sessions
"Psychedelics, Therapy, and Society"
    (summit), 185
psychological domain
  challenging experiences during psychedelic
    sessions and, 137, 142–147
  preparation sessions and, 101, 102–103

psycholytic, defined, 46
PTSD (post-traumatic stress disorder) treatment, 20, 25, 29, 33, 161

Rasmusson, Calle, 108
reconnection, psychedelic psychotherapy and, 184–185
recreational uses of psychedelics, 34, 37–38
reflection and writing exercises, ancestral domain and, 104–105
reflection phase of integration, 201–202
reflection prompts, 201–202
religious context, aligning with core values and growing up in, 77–78. *See also* spirituality
repetition, practice and, 205, 206, 209
retreats, 132–135
    preparation process, 97
    for special operations veterans, 179–183
    vetting, 132
Rice, Nykol Bailey, 6–8, 140–141
Richards, Bill, 175–176

Sacred Knowledge (Richards), 176
safety within psychedelic sessions, 155–159
sangha/satsang, 207
secrets, revealed/shared in psychedelic state, 46–48, 144–147, 176
self
    expanded sense of cosmic, 174–176
    knowing the whole, 166–167
self-acceptance, psychedelic medicine and increase in, 9
self-blame, confronting during psychedelic session, 143
self-care, 4, 131–132
self-hatred/self-loathing, 51–52, 59
self-love, 12, 18, 70–74, 208–209
self-perception, changing, 74
self-reported subjective data, in psychedelic neuroscience research, 8–9
self-worth, 9, 59
serotonin, psychedelics and, 7, 29, 33

serotonin syndrome, 5-MeO-DMT and risk of, 28
sexuality, embodying, 171–173
shadow parts, 165
shamans, 39
Shimodaira, Kenya, 28
signs, subconscious speaking in, 128–129
Smith, Huston, 176
Socratic questioning, 134
somatic awareness during psychedelic session, 128
somatic domain, challenging experiences during psychedelic sessions and, 137, 140–142. *See also* physiological domain
Somatic Experiencing (SE), 15
soundbath, healing, 134
spiritual beliefs, 103–104, 147, 149–150, 157
spiritual domain
    challenging experiences during psychedelic sessions and, 137, 139, 147–152
    preparation sessions and, 101, 103–104
spiritual effects of psychedelic medicines, 10–15
Spiritual Emergency (Grof & Grof), 200
spiritual/spirituality
    daily practices, 104
    what it means to be, 221
spiritual truths, 48
Stein, Steve, 185–186
Stevens, Calvin, 34
StreetSmart Wisdom (podcast), 185
support system, for integration phase, 199, 202–205
surrender, COST stance and, 112–113
Suzuki, Shunryu, 72
symbols
    role in healing and transformation, 164, 167–169
    subconscious speaking in, 128–129

Tao Te Ching (Taoism), 221
Taylor, Kylea, 99

Telomere Effect (Blackburn & Epel), 216–217
temple
    preparing to enter, 116–117
    stepping inside, 118–119
therapeutic exploration phase, of psychedelic session, 124–128
therapeutic goals, 95
therapeutic uses of psychedelics, 40–41
therapist
    bearing witness and, 159–161
    challenging experiences during psychedelic sessions and, 136–137, 139
    dealing with client's difficulty handling ego dissolution, 148–150
    ethical obligations, 152–153
    exploratory questions during psychedelic session, 124–125
    helping client face unwelcomed presence during session, 151
    as mandated reporters, 146–147
    preparing client, 95
    role in psychedelic psychotherapy, 41–43
    roles during psychedelic sessions, 124–125, 127
    safety during sessions and, 155–159
therapist-client relationship and, 98–99, 152–154, 159–161
Traditional Chinese Medicine, 141
traditional healers, 39
traditional therapy, psychedelic therapy *vs.*, 4
training, therapeutic journey as, 219
transference, 153
transformation
    dependent on individual rather than psychedelic, 43–44
    psychedelic sessions and, 135
    truth and, 48–50
transformational practice, 209–210. *See also* practice
trauma
    affecting and changing the body, 83
    inherited, 104
    intergenerational, 3, 104
    reconnecting to joy, 184
    responses to, 64
trust
    building, 118–119
    between client and healer, 98–99
    COST stance and, 114
truth
    arising during psychedelic psychotherapy process, 121–122
    defining, 48–50
    as medicine for patchwork persona, 66–68
    power of, 46–48
    speaking one's, 5, 12
    types of, 48–49
    universal, 48, 50

unconscious, Jung on, 166
universal truths, 48, 50
"Until One Is Committed" (Murray), 79–80
uses of psychedelics, 37–43
    ceremonial, 38–40
    psychotherapeutic, 41–43
    recreational, 34, 37–38
    therapeutic (inner-directed), 40–41

values, integration and clarifying your, 202–205
van der Kolk, Bessel, 83
Vieten, Cassandra, 81, 203, 204–205, 206, 209–210
visions, role in healing and transformation, 164
vomiting, during psychedelic session, 138–139

Warren, Frank, 46–47, 145
"welcome the unwelcome," 139
wisdom, 19
    aligning with, 78–79
    contained within the body, 84–85
Wood Brothers, 181
World Health Organization, 39

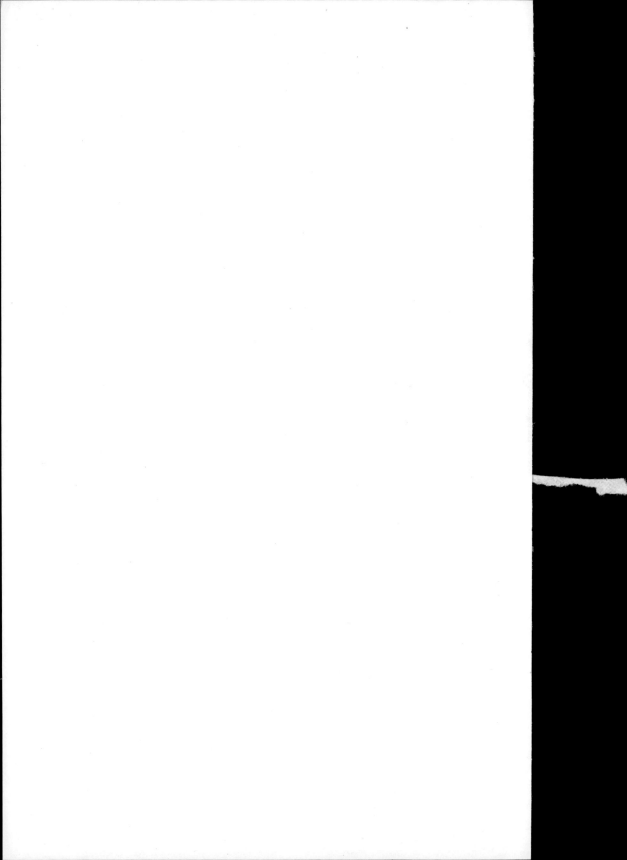